# Wave Your Fat Goodbye

Robert & Lori Evans

# Wave Your Fat *Goodbye*

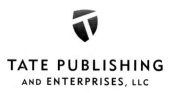

TATE PUBLISHING
AND ENTERPRISES, LLC

Published by Tate Publishing & Enterprises, LLC
127 E. Trade Center Terrace | Mustang, Oklahoma 73064 USA
1.888.361.9473 | www.tatepublishing.com

Tate Publishing is committed to excellence in the publishing industry. The company reflects the philosophy established by the founders, based on Psalm 68:11,
*"The Lord gave the word and great was the company of those who published it."*

Book design copyright © 2013 by Tate Publishing, LLC. All rights reserved.
*Cover design by Joel Uber*
*Interior design by Jomel Pepito*

Published in the United States of America

ISBN: 978-1-62510-408-3
1. Health & Fitness / Diet & Nutrition / Weight Loss
2. Health & Fitness / Healthy Living
13.04.04

# Table of Contents

# Foreword

*A*pproximately 80 million Americans will go on a diet this year, trapped in a seemingly endless cycle spent searching for a magic recipe that will finally work for them.

The *weight* is over. You can finally *Wave Your Fat Goodbye* for good! This ultimate weight loss handbook offers the perfect mixture of humor and simple how-to lessons that will work and last. You will marvel at the fact that all this time your hands have held the key to staying healthy and that God has given you the tools to a better life. It's not about a diet, the latest fad, or cutting certain food groups from your meals; it's about controlling your portion sizes and sowing healthy seed into your body to make permanent changes and live a healthier life. It's time to get the results that you have always wanted so that you can tell everyone that you have finally found *it* and you are *Waving Your Fat Goodbye.*

# Introduction

*F*or the past several years we've been blessed to write, produce and host the Christian Fitness television show and interact with viewers from all over the country. They've shared their frustrations with us about yo-yo dieting or their inability to follow strict meal plans and strenuous workout routines. The quality of their lives has suffered because of the negative toll that an unhealthy lifestyle has placed on their bodies. These stories are what inspired a desire in us to write this book and outline a simple approach to help readers, like you, make lasting changes in their lives. We wanted to offer a solution that would guide you through an uncomplicated course that includes a basic starting point and then walks you through easy-to-follow tips on how to stay on track. To get you to a place where you can stop unjustly blaming the washing machine for shrinking your clothes and recognize that it has been a few poor decisions that have caused your clothes to fit tighter. To realize that we all bear the fruit of the seed that we plant and fast food restaurants and donuts are not the best seed to yield a healthy harvest. There are hundreds of different seeds out there that you can plant in your field, but what is the harvest of each one?

So you want to lose weight and be healthier, right? Fantastic! Reaching your goal is as easy as following a simple God-given tool and waving off your fat. You have the power in your hands to control and maintain the ultimate healthy weight that is just right for you, but it's not only in your hands, a lot of it depends on your head. That little bit of matter between your ears is what really matters. Disciplining your mind by educating yourself on healthier choices and portion control will give you the tools that will help you to make changes today that will last for a lifetime.

So if you're ready to get started, the first thing you need to do is to speak this out as loud as you can. "*I will start sowing the right seed for a healthy harvest!*" Go ahead. Wherever you are, right now, regardless of who is around; say this out loud, "I will start sowing the right seed for a healthy harvest!"

Did we have you do that as a verbal commitment or positive reinforcement through cognitive action? No. It was just an exercise to see if you are truly willing to take a chance and step out of the boat in order to change your life. Plus, if anyone was around and heard you then you most likely embarrassed yourself to such an extreme that the rest of your journey will be fairly simple in comparison. It will be a "piece of cake"; as "easy as pie." Where did those sayings come from anyway? Your goal is to live a healthier life but even subliminal comments like those have crept into our everyday language, causing us to constantly talk about foods that we should avoid. That's just a precursor to the obstacles that you'll face throughout your journey, but once you learn to recognize and conquer them, the victory will be yours.

Do you remember the old saying you are what you eat? We'll you're not only what you eat, but you are also what you speak as well. We're going to guide you through several series on how to eat properly but we also want to encourage you to speak healthy. Speak and profess the right things over your life and your new journey to living healthier. The words that come out of your mouth have incredible power, so try to speak positive things over your life. If you don't believe us, then let's ask God what He has to say about it? "Death and life are in the power of the tongue, and they who indulge in it shall eat the fruit of it [for death or life]" (Proverbs 18:21 AMP).

There are really only two things that you need to be successful in your journey to living a healthier life: your brain and the Word of God. Use scripture to reinforce and remind yourself to keep your mind refreshed and renewed and don't be afraid to deny your body the sugar that your mind is tempting you into thinking that you need. "We are destroying speculations and every lofty thing raised up against the knowledge of God, and we are taking every thought captive to the obedience of Christ" (2 Corinthians 10:5 NASB).

Write this 2nd Corinthian verse down on a post it note and place it on your bathroom mirror or on the dashboard of your car and remind yourself to "take every thought captive." When you think about eating the wrong foods, take that thought captive. When you take something captive it no longer has control. As your captive thought you now control it so simply tell that thought of having a donut, "no, I will not allow you to enter my mind, so go now and never return." That's how you speak to a captive thought, you don't allow it to get out and you definitely don't act upon it.

The same goes for Galatians 5:24 (NKJV) which says "and those who are Christ's have crucified the flesh with its passions and desires."

When your body starts craving sugar, deny it that desire and replace it with something healthy. Scripture and the simple power that you hold within your own hands are the tools you'll need as we teach you how to start living the healthier and more productive life that God has planned for you. So get ready to *start sowing the right seed for a healthy harvest*!

# Facing Your Obstacles

*B*efore we jump right into the kitchen with Lori and detail portion sizes for you, one of the first steps that you want to take is to recognize some of the obstacles that are currently preventing you from achieving your ultimate health. Here is a list of roadblocks. See if any of them sound familiar or ring true for you.

- Repetition–I always go down isle #8 and grab two 12 packs of soda, right before I get milk and eggs.

- Routine – Every Friday after school I take the kids for some drive-thru fast food. They love it.

- Temptation & Your Mind – I can't resist grabbing some Doritos at the grocery store. It's almost as if they call out to me by name.

- Comfort – When I'm home alone or upset I tend to find myself raiding the cabinets.

- Snacks & Sweets – But it's my third cousin, twice removed, on my Godmother's side of the

family's Birthday. It only comes around once
a year.

- Taste – Low fat and fat free foods are tasteless
  and boring. Plus, my mother raised me to have
  great taste.

- Not Enough Time – I don't have time to cook
  let alone time to shop for healthy foods.

- I Can't Afford It – Fast food is so inexpensive I
  can't afford to shop on my own and buy fresh.

- Sin – I know I shouldn't eat it, but a few bites
  won't hurt me.

These are just a few of the obstacles that might have
contributed to you adopting an unhealthy lifestyle, but
you can overcome every one of them and we're going
to show you how. Later in the book we're going to
give you all of the tools to make permanent changes
through proper portion sizes, but it's imperative that
you recognize where you might stumble, and learn
to overcome these obstacles by altering a few habits
that will then help you change not just your life, but
your lifestyle.

Remember your pledge; *I will start sowing the right
seed for a healthy harvest*! Your body is like a field (don't
take offense to that statement, it's meant as a metaphor).
If you were a farmer and wanted to grow turnips, then
you would plant turnip seeds. If you wanted to yield a
harvest of soy beans, then you have to plant soy beans.

So you get the metaphor, right? Sow the seed for the harvest that you want to receive.

Start by considering yourself the farmer of your own body (if you picture yourself in overalls, holding a pitchfork, with a piece of hay in your mouth, this mental exercise will be a lot more fun). You want to be healthy so you need to be concerned about every single seed that you plant in your body. If a farmer wants turnips but isn't really paying attention and just throws whatever seeds he can find into the row, then the few turnip seeds that may have been included will end up loosing the nutrients that they need to another more aggressive crop. Or if he doesn't tend to the field then weeds can strangle the harvest. Treat your body the exact same way that you would treat your field. Just because you ate an apple and had some oatmeal for breakfast doesn't mean that you can eat pizza and fries for lunch and dinner. Everything that you plant will have a harvest. If you plant donuts and French fries, then your harvest will be a donut around your waist, French fry thighs, and clogged arteries. If you plant the right portions of fruits and vegetables, then your harvest will be a healthy and strong body.

You can come in out of the field now and put your pitchfork away, we're going to go back and address some of the obstacles that you might face and educate you on how to overcome them. It's vital that you understand and acknowledge areas where you might stumble; educate yourself, and then avoid those pitfalls. The Word of God reminds us to seek understanding and wisdom. "The beginning of wisdom is: Acquire wisdom; And with all your acquiring, get understanding" (Proverbs 4:7 NASB).

# Repetition

We'll start with the first obstacle, *repetition*. It's easy to make a few poor choices each day, and many of them are just out of habit from repetition. It can seem as harmless as adding 3 tablespoons of sugar to your coffee every morning or as flagrant as believing that you have to have dessert or something sweet every night after dinner. Some research suggests that it takes 21 days to break a bad habit or to form a new one, but there is more compelling research that pushes that number closer to 66 days.[1] In order to break that bad habit, we want you to think about the effect it will have on your field (your body)? For every single liquid or solid that you pick up at the grocery store or put into your mouth for the next 66 days (and beyond that), think of it as a seed. What kind of a harvest is it going to yield? We'll reference our earlier example of *going down isle #8 and grabbing two 12 packs of soda*. The bottled water is usually right next to the soda in the grocery store, so instead of reaching for the soda, load up the bottom of your cart with water or buy a filtered water pitcher and save tons of money. If you add up how much you spend on soda versus replacing a water filter every month, you wind up saving a small fortune.

What would you rather put into your field anyway, soda or water? Imagine what soda would do to a row of turnip seeds? Water will cause them to prosper, grow and flourish. Soda takes oil stains off of your driveway and corrosion off of your car battery leads, so why would you want that in your stomach anyway? Because it tastes better? We'll cover taste in a later chapter so keep reading, but if you avoid soda for our recommendation of 66 days and then drink some, it will taste so sweet that you'll instantly realize how detrimental it is to your field.

# Routine

*A* close relative to repetition is *routine*. We get so accustomed to performing a certain task at the same time or during a certain event that it becomes second nature and we don't even think about it anymore, we just do it on autopilot. We mentioned earlier; *every Friday after school I take the kids for some drive-thru fast food. They love it.*

In order to change a routine you need to change the environment. The example of fast food that we used is a tough one because you're competing against restaurants that spend a fortune targeting and enticing children with advertising and toys, so you need to be creative and develop a new routine that is healthier but still fun. One of our suggestions is to drop by the grocery store instead of fast food and let your children pick whatever fruit and vegetable they want. Encourage them to try something different every few weeks. It might be a star fruit, some cantaloupe, or try a different berry each week this month: strawberry, raspberry, blueberry & blackberries. Have them go on the computer and research all of the different types of tomatoes and then see which kinds they can find at your grocery store. It can become a fun hunting adventure for them. They will become more educated about different healthy foods and that can last a lifetime. The first few weeks might be tough to compete against the toys offered by the clown and the king, but the attitude of our children can often be a reflection of our own attitude. If you make it an event filled with fun and laughter; that attitude will be contagious and you'll be able to pass along that joy to your children and create wonderful memories. This isn't limited to just children. Even if you are single and shopping on your own, you can still do the research and go on a grocery store scavenger hunt. People spend hours on the internet playing farm games, well why not spend a little time participating in a real farm game, tending to your own field!

Change the environment and you can change your routines. You can also apply this principle to the routine of sitting on the couch for hours every night. A simple walk around the block is a change of environment and can create a fantastic healthy new routine for everyone involved and create fond memories for a lifetime. When Lori was young, she would spend her summers in Miami with her grandparents and they would go for walks and talk every night after dinner. Those are some of her most precious memories of their time together. Something as simple as spending time together can have a lasting impact.

To show you how dangerous routines can be we're going to present you with an example of eating at your favorite restaurant. If you're accustomed to ordering unhealthy items when you eat out without thinking about it, then we want to encourage you to think about it and change your routine. A few simple wrong decisions when ordering your meal can have enormous effects, and we do mean enormous. You can easily consume five times the calories that you should in just one meal. If your only course is a healthy salad then you're probably okay but the normal meal at a restaurant will feature three to five separate courses.

Let's start with one of the first things that you encounter: your drink. The wrong decision would be a soda. That's 200 calories, 20 milligrams of sodium, 52 grams of carbohydrates and 52 grams of sugar. The right choice would be water. You just saved 200 calories and 52 grams of sugar. That's more than a 200 percent savings on your calories. If you're a parent then bypassing soda is also teaching your children that water is a healthier choice and that will become their routine as they get older. Here's a quick fact to reinforce choosing water. Your brain consists of around 70-80% water, so hydrate it the proper way. Most brains contain 0% percent soda so wouldn't water be the logical choice?

The next hurdle at the restaurant is the basket of bread that they bring to the table. French and Italian bread have almost double the calories, two times as much sodium, and twice as many carbohydrates as rye bread. And you probably don't eat your bread dry, you'll want to dip it into olive oil (120 calories) or add some butter (100 calories). So two pieces of Italian bread with olive oil is 426 calories and you haven't even started your salad yet. If you just nibbled on one piece of rye bread you could save 385 calories.

Next up is your salad. The wrong choice would be a tossed salad with avocado, walnuts, a hard boiled egg, shredded cheese, bacon bits and ranch dressing. This simple salad is a whopping 873 calories. The right choice would be a spinach salad with cherry tomatoes, cucumber, carrots and a low fat Italian dressing. That's only 144 calories so your savings are another 729 calories.

Now for the main course. We're going to have 3 ounces of fish tonight. The wrong choice is fried with tartar sauce; that's 448 calories compared to only 350 calories for grilled fish with some lemon.

What about the side dishes? We choose to have broccoli and mashed potatoes. Steamed broccoli with a little lemon is only 12 calories and plain mashed potatoes are only 90. Now the wrong choice; broccoli with salt and cheese is 180 calories and mashed potatoes with butter and gravy is 720 calories.

Finally; what would eating out be without dessert. If you eat an entire piece of pie then you can add another 200 calories. Our advice is to share one piece with the entire table and then your two bites is only about 30 calories.

If we total up your meal, here is the difference:

| Dinner Item | Dangerous Routine | # calories | | Healthier Alternative | # calories | Difference |
|---|---|---|---|---|---|---|
| drink | soda | 200 | vs. | water | 0 | -200 |
| bread | French bread w/ /oil | 426 | vs. | rye | 41 | -385 |
| salad | chef salad | 873 | vs. | spinach | 144 | -729 |
| fish | fried fish | 448 | vs. | grilled fish | 350 | -98 |
| side dish broccoli | w/ cheese | 180 | vs. | w/ lemon | 12 | -168 |
| side dish of potato | seasoning & gravy | 720 | vs. | plain mashed | 90 | -630 |
| dessert | piece of pie | 200 | vs. | 2 bites of pie | 30 | -170 |
| TOTAL | | 3,047 | | | 667 | -2,380 |

The total calorie count for the dangerous routine meal is 3,047. The healthier alternative meal is only 667 calories. A total difference in just this one meal is 2,380 calories. That's more calories than most people should consume in an entire day. So the synopsis of our little exercise is to change your routine by making quality decisions.

# Temptation and Your Mind

*B*y changing your environment you can change your repetition and routines. The same goes for *temptations* that you might encounter. It's imperative that you guard your eyes and ears as much as possible and construct a new mindset toward whatever item seems irresistible to you. Change your environment whenever possible to avoid certain foods that cause temptation. If hot fudge sundaes are your weakness, then don't go to an ice cream shop after a Little League game; choose an establishment that offers yogurt and fruit instead. Don't go to the movie theater if you can't control yourself. If the allure of the snack counter is too strong, then watch a movie at home.

Our earlier example of one of the obstacles that you might face was: *I can't resist grabbing some Doritos at the grocery store.* The first thing that you need to do is remember to take your thoughts captive. We make decisions every second of every day of our lives, so choose the correct path. You've learned discipline in more areas than you might realize, and the irresistible food at the grocery store is just one more that you have to conquer. Think about how many instantaneous decisions you make throughout the day, starting the very second that you awaken. As soon as the alarm goes off in the morning you are confronted with a path of choices; to get up or hit the snooze button? Then the decisions begin to multiply at a rapid pace; to wash your hair or not, shave your legs or not (not much of a decision for men unless you're a competitive swimmer). What to wear, what to feed the kids, etc....

You are faced with that same path of decisions and temptation when you come up on the aisle with Doritos at the grocery store. We don't mean to single out Doritos, but they are incredibly hard to resist and they aren't one of the top ten healthiest snacks. One vending machine size 50gram bag has 250 calories with 120 of those calories coming from fat. In defense of Doritos, they do make a baked nacho cheese chip that is much lower in calories. They are still full of sodium and have almost no nutritional value, but at least they are making a lower calorie version. Since we're talking about temptation, think about this fact for a moment; they have one flavor called blazin' and they come in a red bag. Doesn't that sound like a representation of a temptation from Satan? We're just throwing that out there as something to ponder.

So you've come to that path in the road at the grocery store. You can choose to go left and grab that bag of chips that has had a stronghold on you, or swerve your cart to the right, away from the temptation. We recommend veering your cart in the opposite direction so hard that you come up on two wheels and as you speed away look back over your shoulder and laugh out loud as you yell, "*you will not conquer me. I will start sowing the right seed for a healthy harvest!*"

Now that you've been kicked out of two grocery stores for causing a scene by yelling at the food and racing around the store (although you've gained a new respect from your kids who now think you're so cool), there is another option that we want to present. We must warn you, this one is not for the faint of heart or someone with a weak stomach, although if you're used to drinking sodas and eating chips then your stomach wall must be like an iron fortress anyway. Think back to a time in your life when you had an experience with food that was so awful that it made you sick. Maybe it was food poisoning and you haven't been able to eat that item ever since. If you've never had such an experience then you are truly blessed. When Robert was a child he couldn't stand eating German potatoes and there was one occasion that they didn't stay down, although they didn't look much different after they came up (okay, that was totally uncalled for and we apologize, but it will help us make our point). Robert can't stand the smell of German potatoes still to this day. He gags if he gets near the smell. If you have experienced such a tragedy, then place that same memory of what we'll call your "yuck" food onto the one item that you simply can't resist. Envision that those irresistible chips look exactly like German potatoes or perhaps those oysters that you got food poisoning from. So the next time that you see chips in the aisle at the grocery store, bring up a mental image of your "yuck" food and you shouldn't have any trouble passing them by. There is no way Robert would put German potatoes from the deli into his shopping cart, and now that he envisions German potatoes every time he sees Doritos, there is no way that Doritos are going to wind up in the cart either.

If you don't think that envisioning your "yuck" food will work, we have one last option, but we must warn you, do not read the remainder of this chapter unless you've exhausted every other technique imaginable. Okay, you've been warned, if you're that desperate; then proceed.

*Warning!* This next part is really disgusting, but true.

(Lori, the co-author, doesn't like to even read this section.)

The FDA (U.S. Food and Drug Administration) actually has a handbook that lists the allowable amounts of mold, insect parts, rodent hairs, larvae, mites, and various other items of what they define as "natural or unavoidable defects in food." For our example we're going to use canned and dried mushrooms. For every 15 grams of dried mushrooms, they are allowed to have 20 or more maggots of any size including 5 or more that are 2mm or longer. Peanut Butter is allowed to have 1 rodent hair per 100 grams. So we want you to make that one food that you can't seem to resist your new "yuck" food by visualizing it filled with one of those "unavoidable defects." Close your eyes for a few seconds and visualize that image. Now do it again two more times imagining a rodent hair or maggot as the dip of choice on top of your chip. We know that this is incredibly gross but we warned you that this was only an option if you weren't able to take every thought captive and control your urge to eat unhealthy items. Now every time that you pass your temptation food at the grocery store or someone offers you some at a luncheon or pot-luck, visualize that "unavoidable defect" image and try to smile as you respectfully decline to partake.

Excerpts from the FDA "Defect Levels Handbook"

| MUSHROOMS, CANNED AND DRIED | Insects (AOAC 967.24) | Average of over 20 or more maggots of any size per 100 grams of drained mushrooms and proportionate liquid or 15 grams of dried mushrooms OR Average of 5 or more maggots 2 mm or longer per 100 grams of drained mushrooms and proportionate liquid or 15 grams of dried mushrooms |
| | Mites (AOAC 967.24) | Average of 75 mites per 100 grams drained mushrooms and proportionate liquid or 15 grams of dried mushrooms |

DEFECT SOURCE: Insects - preharvest insect infestation, Mites - preharvest and/or post harvest infestation, Decomposition - preharvest infection

| PEANUT BUTTER | Insect filth (AOAC 968.35) | Average of 30 or more insect fragments per 100 grams |
| | Rodent filth (AOAC 968.35) | Average of 1 or more rodent hairs per 100 grams |

DEFECT SOURCE: Insect fragments - preharvest and/or post harvest and/or processing insect infestation, Rodent hair - post harvest and/or processing contamination with animal hair or excreta.

(source-http://www.fda.gov/food/guidancecomplianceregulatoryinformation/guidancedocuments/sanitation/ucm056174.htm)

# Comfort

nother obstacle to reaching your healthy weight goal is to understand how, when and why you stumble. Many of us don't even realize it but we turn to food for *comfort*. It can be as a reaction to an emotional event or often times just from simple boredom. Have you ever found yourself raiding the cabinets or going through an entire ice cream container when you were upset? Or you aren't able to watch a movie without having a bag of popcorn, a candy bar or some Good & Plenty's. If you don't feel as though you can control your urges, then educate yourself on healthier alternatives and use them as replacements when you absolutely have to have your comfort food. There's nothing wrong with having some popcorn during a movie, but skip the butter, salt, and cheese, and try to eat air popped instead of oil cooked. Air popped is only 31 calories with just 3 calories from fat, versus 64 calories with 43 calories from fat for oil popped, and 170 calories with 108 calories from fat if you add butter.

You can use these same principles for ice cream. A half cup of rich vanilla ice cream is 266 calories with

156 from fat. So try low-fat yogurt instead. Light N' Fit has a 6 ounce version that is only 80 calories with 0 from fat. We know, you're thinking that it doesn't taste as good but if you're eating out of emotion or boredom, taste isn't really the issue. Plus if you add some fruit to your yogurt it's delicious, much better than vanilla ice cream. Remember your pledge, you are sowing seed, so control your mind and sow healthier seed.

Eating for comfort or out of boredom are dangerous habits to adopt. Think about the farmer scenario again and consider the seed that you are planting. A farmer doesn't sow seed when they are bored or upset, so why would you? Learn to recognize when you're bored and go for a walk instead of needlessly snacking. If you find yourself eating for no apparent reason while watching TV, get your Bible out and open it so that your hands are busy instead of using them to shovel bad seed into your field. If you absolutely have to have a comfort food, think of creative and healthy alternatives. Try freezing some grapes and eating a handful. They are cool, refreshing, and it takes a little while to eat each one so you aren't shoveling dozens of calories down in a short period of time. You can also make your own frozen sickles by freezing other fruits: strawberries, raspberries, even apple slices or banana chips. Have you ever had slices of a banana as frozen chips? They're delicious.

# Snacks

*nacking* can be the downfall for many people that attempt to live a healthier life. They do great at meal times by eating the proper foods, controlling their portion sizes, but those pesky snacks ruin their calorie count and they don't even realize it. What you eat between meals, or even while you're cooking meals, can devastate your harvest. You were doing so well tending to your field and then your snacks come in like a swarm of locust and ruin your crop. Remember that every minute of your life you come to a fork in the road concerning what decision to make. You stop to fill up your car with gas and decide to run in for a drink. You grab a fountain soda and a bag of chips (16ounce drink = 220 calories + 12 chips = 140calories), that's almost 400 calories with no nutritional value and the majority of calories from fat. The other detriment to this behavior is the amount of money that adds up at the end of the month. Keep a log of every single penny that you spend. Write it in a little notebook and look at it at the end of the month. You'll be amazed at how much you spend with just a few quick stops at a coffee shop, a trip or two through the drive through, a snack at the movies, your trip into the store while pumping gas, or the dreaded vending machine at the office. One of the keys to living a healthier life is controlling when, where and what you snack on. Often times you're not even thirsty or hungry, but snack out of routine from past experiences. If you are thirsty, grab bottled water, and for a snack, keep a Tupperware container full of mixed nuts and dried fruits in your car or office desk drawer. One small handful of nuts can curb your appetite for several hours. We also recommend the same guidelines if you're traveling, but on a much larger scale. Pack a small cooler full of healthy wraps, fruits and vegetables. You'll save a fortune by not being tempted to hit the drive through and you'll save some driving time by not stopping as often. If you need to stop and stretch your legs you can now swing into a rest area and enjoy your healthy picnic at a table while enjoying the outdoors. It can add much better memories to the trip than the frustration of trying to order a meal through a speaker that sounds like Charlie Brown's teacher.

Another area of snacking that is often overlooked is how much you sneak while you're cooking. It's easy to try and justify snacking on a few cookies while preparing dinner thinking that it won't hurt you, when in reality those extra and empty calories are hurting you. You just threw garbage into your field. Your body didn't need it because there wasn't any nutritional value; it was just garbage that adds up to polluting the potential harvest of your field. As a farmer would you pour grease into the row of turnip seeds that you just planted? Well that's exactly what you're doing by adding garbage to your own body. Snacking while cooking is like leaking oil from your tractor as you plow your field. You're polluting the row before you even plant your seed.

They used to say "never trust a skinny chef," but we would say just the opposite and encourage you to "trust a healthy chef." Would you take swimming lessons from an adult that has to wear arm floaties; piano lessons from someone that just learned to play "Chopsticks" and can't coordinate both fingers to play at the same time; or what about advice on changing your own car oil from someone that opens your center console to look for the dip stick to check the fluid levels? The Bible tells us to seek Godly wisdom, so take your advice from knowledgeable people. If someone tells you that this is going to taste great and be really healthy for you but you had to duck out of the way of the button that just went whizzing by your head because their pants couldn't take the pressure of their expanding stomach, then you might want to reconsider taking their advice. We don't mean any offense to someone struggling with their weight but refrain from taking their advice until after they've gained a victory in that area. Use wisdom and trust a healthy chef for advice on more nutritious eating.

If you're the chef of your own kitchen you want to be wary of how much you sample or taste test while cooking. There's nothing wrong with testing the amount of spice you need to add by taking a little sip, but when that sip is accompanied by an entire piece of bread dipped into your broth as a taste test, then the calories in those samples will really start to add up. When a small portion of every ingredient makes it into your personal pan (your stomach), then you're defeating your healthy eating plan before you even serve the meal. Even if you don't sample parts of the meal, the aromas during preparation often combine to penetrate your defenses and you surrender by grabbing a cookie or chips to munch on. To avoid snacking while cooking, grab a glass of water and drink it before you even start to get all of your ingredients out for the meal. We even recommend filling your glass up a second time and drinking that as well. The water can help dissipate some of your cravings. You can also cut some celery into small chunks before you start cooking and use that as your snack. The combination of the bulk of the celery and the water will fill you up so that you can resist the temptation.

Snacks aren't part of your daily meals; they're just something to hold you over so that you don't gorge yourself into a food induced comatose state at dinner time. Look for healthy alternatives to keep your harvest plentiful.

Here's a simple list of a few snack alternatives:

| Avoid | # calories | | Alternative | # calories | savings |
|---|---|---|---|---|---|
| donut (refined sugars and trans fats) | 250 | – TRY – | apple (6ounces) | 90 | 160 |
| corn chips (1bag / 7 chips) | 300 | – TRY – | raw almonds (handful of 20) | 20 | 280 |
| potato chips (1 bag) | 300 | – TRY – | baby carrots (6 ounces) | 60 | 240 |
| hot dog (mystery meat) | 240 | – TRY – | 2 slices of low-fat turkey - rolled up | 120 | 120 |
| chicken nuggets (6) | 300 | – TRY – | dried fruit (2ounces) | 130 | 170 |
| yogurt cup (grocery store w/ fruit/corn syrup, 8ounces) | 400 | – TRY – | banana (1medium) | 60 | 340 |
| milk chocolate candy bar | 215 | – TRY – | dark chocolate (1 ounce) | 100 | 115 |
| milk shake | 400 | – TRY – | strawberry / apple smoothie | 200 | 200 |

A lot of the examples above that we encourage you to avoid are empty calories and filled with chemicals to add to the taste or to increase their shelf life. They carry no nutritional value what so ever, so we've given you some alternatives that are natural, God given foods that are half the calories. Your body will thank you for avoiding the chemicals and you will feel so much better, sleep better, and create a healthier you by waving some of your fat goodbye. Many of the chemicals in foods can actually make you sick over time, so educate yourself through research and come up with some of your own healthy snack alternatives.

# Taste

One of the battles that many people face is that unhealthy foods taste so incredibly good. The sweeteners and sugar are like a drug. Cupcakes and cookies are like candy crack. You're trying to eat healthier and someone offers you a thin mint cookie. Isn't that an oxymoron? It might be a thin cookie but since it's covered in chocolate they might want to rename it a "thin mint fattener." When you see that irresistible cookie, remember this one simple phrase; *sugar is evil!* New research suggests that sugar is linked to inflammation in the body that results in premature aging, loss of skin elasticity, wrinkles and various other pains and misery.

We don't mean to speak out against that certain mint cookie or try to denigrate organizations that have fund raisers and sell such items. Most of those groups are phenomenal for children and help to build tomorrow's leaders, but they do tempt you with unhealthy food choices but that's because they sell what people will buy. You can always just bless an organization by donating a few dollars and let them keep the food. You don't have to buy cookies or a hot dog, just give them a few dollars.

You saved that money by not buying sodas last week anyway, so help someone else out. Remember your commitment to start waving your fat goodbye so don't kid yourself and think that you can control yourself once you open that sleeve of cookies. Don't allow them into your home at all and then you can celebrate your victory over temptation. Simple little battles like this one that will help you stay on track and realize your goal. Keep a mental log of this victory, or write it down if you need to, and remember it the next time you are tempted so you know that you've beaten it before and can do so again.

Let's get off of that rabbit trail about sugar and get back to taste (if you don't know what that comment means, a rabbit trail is when someone gets sidetracked in thought and goes down a completely different trail than their original focus). A key that we want to concentrate on to help you with your healthier eating is to find and create recipes that taste good. You don't have to have sugars and sweets to improve the taste of a meal. There are several methods to reduce your dependency on sweet tasting foods and we like to use milk as a prime example. Whole milk is loaded with fat and really shouldn't be consumed after around 2 years of age. It is much healthier to drink fat free, skim milk, or 2%, but taste is a major issue here. If you are accustomed to drinking regular milk it might take a little while to wean yourself from it. If you go from regular vitamin D milk and start drinking fat free, at first it will taste like cheap, flavored water. You'll think that you'll never be able to get accustomed to it, but stay with it. Continue to drink fat free for at least 2 months, and that includes if you add any to your coffee. After 2 months we would encourage you to have a little sample of regular vitamin D milk again. In most studies the participants have acknowledged that after about two months of drinking reduced fat milk that regular milk now tastes like they're drinking pure cream and is almost too much to handle. Your taste buds will have adapted to the fat free and that will now become your new routine. If it doesn't work after 2 months, try 6 months. If you're still having trouble adjusting to the lower fat content, then just think about your commitment to sowing seed and keep pushing through. If you're still struggling after 6 months then try it for 20 years (hee hee, seriously, the Bible talks about growing up and not drinking milk any longer, of course that's spiritual maturity but the same can apply to your food choices). If you're still struggling after 20 years then you have larger issues than just the taste of milk and might need some serious prayer (we don't want to offend anyone with that statement, but seriously, it's just a slight taste difference, so do yourself a favor and just commit to changing).

Your taste buds can and will adapt to new and different foods and tastes. You don't have to continue to use the same additives and condiments that you grew up with. Some of the biggest culprits that add extra calories to your meal are butter, creams, salt and sauces. Take a baked potato for example; skip the butter, sour cream and cheese and try adding salsa, vegetables, or olive oil and herbs. With that one simple step you can reduce the calorie count for your baked potato to less than one third. The right amount of salsa on a baked potato can be delicious so you don't have to sacrifice taste you just have to be creative.

Sure, it sounds simple for a baked potato but what about fish, turkey or chicken? You can apply the same principles that we outlined for drinking milk to your protein as well.

When preparing your wild caught fish or free range lean turkey and chicken, make sure that you bake or broil it, never eat it fried, and avoid the fattening sauces and marinades. Try some of the same condiments that we mentioned for your baked potato; salsa, vegetables, and marinade and bake your poultry with herbs, either fresh or dried. Create your flavors with herbs instead of sauces. The natural flavors of the meat will come to life when you just heighten it with herbs, which are God's natural flavorings anyway. Quit hiding the taste of your food behind creams and sauces because they tend to overpower and dominate the flavor. Try experimenting with herbs. The next time your church is having a bake sale or a pot-luck lunch, be creative and offer something healthy that you flavored with herbs. Encourage everyone else to experiment and then you can share tips with each other and start adopting an environment of creating a healthier congregation. You can still use the recipe that has been handed down for generations, just substitute some of the ingredients and you can leave a new and healthier legacy for the generations to come.

# Not Enough Time

What is the one thing that you can't turn back? Time. You can turn a clock back and change the time, but that doesn't take you back. When we were younger we couldn't wait to get older and as we get older we wish we were younger. Hollywood can make creative and clever movies with DeLoreans. Ponce De Leon can search the wilds for a fountain, and scientists can propose theories on wormholes and the ability to bend time and space, but none of them has been able to get back even one second of their lives. The only hope that we have is to spend the time that we do have as wisely as possible, and that means making time to live healthier.

We are all so busy these days that there never seems to be enough time to get everything accomplished, let alone take the time to shop for healthier foods or spend time cooking. We want to encourage you to *make time*. Step back for just a moment and take a look at your life; reevaluate what is really important to you and your family. Is it imperative that your children be in dance, little league baseball, pottery class, tennis lessons, swim class, and cub scouts all just on Tuesday evening? Use the same notepad that we mentioned earlier to write down your monthly miscellaneous expenses on and write down how much time you spend each day doing different functions. You might be surprised to learn that you watch 4 hours of TV every night or that it takes you 3 hours to get ready in the morning because you're watching the news, updating Facebook online, or trying on 6 different outfits even though you wind up always wearing the very first outfit anyway.

So where can you save some time? Did you write in your memo pad that it took you 10 minutes to drive to a fast food restaurant the other night, and then you spent another 5 minutes in line ordering, another 10 minutes to drive back home, then 15 minutes to sit in front of the TV and eat. So you spent 40 minutes for "fast food" which in this case would be more appropriately called "lazy food." In those 40 minutes you could have easily prepared a much healthier meal at home and probably in less time.

Or what about the other night when you were tired and didn't feel like cooking so you ordered pizza delivery? You were still willing to wait over 30 minutes for someone to bring you your diner and then you'll tip them because you were too lazy (that word might be a bit strong, let us rephrase that), you're too inundated with the distractions of everyday life to spend those 30 minutes cooking some noodles and getting out a jar of marinara sauce. Don't get us wrong. We're all for the convenience of fast food (healthy fast food like apples) or a special pizza delivery treat on a Friday Movie Night, but they should never become the norm. It's pretty common knowledge how unhealthy the majority of fast food is, so we want to encourage you to start making time to enjoy normal meals cooked at home; colorful, well-balanced, and healthy choices.

There are television networks, magazines, books, and even internet sites that are all dedicated solely to recipes and cooking. Several have broken it down and tailored their focus to emphasizing a preparation time of 30 minutes or less for the entire meal. So spend a little time shopping or surfing the internet and start a recipe collection of your own. You remember, the kind of recipe box that your mother or grandmother used to have sitting on the kitchen counter. Start one of your own and get the entire family involved in keeping it up to date and current.

We encourage you to turn your priority clock back to the days of old when families actually cooked and prepared the meal together, helped each other set the table, then sat down and prayed over the food and ate a good healthy meal while having actual conversations with each other. It was a family dinner table with no interruptions by cell phones, no children texting their friends, no earphones blasting favorite IPod tunes, no TV captivating everyone's attention. It was a discussion about life, the Bible, politics, and ideas. It was a time for families to think, grow, and actually be a family.

So if you're picking up your meals from a clown, a king or a redheaded freckle faced girl more than once every few weeks, then you're inviting more than just unhealthy physical troubles into your home! You might be on the road to a future where you will look back and say, "I wish I would have done… (insert your own potential or actual regret here)." If you haven't done so already, start making changes today.

You will undoubtedly have to make some sacrifices in order to free up additional time for cooking and spending time together as a family or couple, but are they really sacrifices or just a change in routine? If you look at the little memo pad that you've been writing the details of how you spend your time, it will reveal quite a bit, especially if you're honest with yourself. Is it really necessary to listen to 2 hours of news each day? We want to stay up to date on current affairs but you can do that in 5 minutes and then spend time at your dinner table discussing some of your own thoughts and ideas on taxes and the economy instead of listening to someone else's opinion for 2 hours. Is it necessary to sit on the couch for three hours every night because you're exhausted from the day's work? Imagine what you could have accomplished or the incredible meal that you could have cooked instead of watching that program that did nothing but try and brainwash you into accepting immorality as a way of life.

Another aspect of time that can help you to live a healthier life is to take your time while eating. Despite what your stomach might tell you, it is not a race to finish your food. If you came from a family with eight siblings then you might dispute that because speed was your only hope of getting your fair share, but we're talking to the other 99 percent of families that need to take their time.

According to a report in Penn Metabolic & Bariatric Surgery News, it takes roughly 20 minutes for the brain and stomach to register fullness.[3] Most of us eat our entire meal in less than 20 minutes so we're cramming so much food into our mouths that our stomach never has time to signal our brain to stop. There is a simple rule that we want you to consider adopting; put your fork down after every single bite. We say fork but it applies to your spoon, knife, fingers, whatever utensil or means of transport you're using to get your food into your mouth. Start a habit of placing your sandwich back on the plate after each bite. You don't need to hold your fork like a ping-pong paddle and use it to speed shovel your green beans in as if you're digging for buried treasure. Hold your fork lightly between your thumb (pollex) and middle finger (digitus me'dius) and apply minimal pressure with your index finger (Digitus Secundus Manus) to slowly maneuver a green bean into your mouth and then place the fork gingerly back onto your plate after that bite and return your hands to your lap while you chew the beans with your lips closed together so that your not showing the entire table your teeth grinding up the beans. If your mouth is open while chewing we would call that *see food*, and generally not something everyone else really wants to see.

Wow, did we really go down another bunny trail and have an etiquette lesson right in the middle of a book on eating healthier? Yes we did, but as Christians, it's important that we be an example of Christ in everything that we do including our table manners. We are to be in the world but not part of the world. It seems that the decline of morals and respect for others is making the world a darker place, more barbaric and less focused on being proper and pure. So be an example to others in all aspects of your life, shining the light of Jesus in all ways.

Now we've gone from an etiquette lesson to some preaching and you're wondering when we'll get back to waving your fat goodbye? We want you to have victory in all areas of your life so we wanted to show you that slowing down your eating can have more impact than just preventing overeating by giving your stomach time to signal that it's full. It can also create an environment of better table manners and an opportunity for you to have conversation and fellowship.

Okay, we're back on track now and ready to continue talking about spending time more wisely. We've covered spending more time with family and less time just being busy, but we also want you to be more prudent during your meal time. When eating, put your fork or utensil down and actually chew your food, enjoy the flavor and taste. Sometimes we eat so fast that our taste buds barely have a chance to enjoy the flavor before we're piling in another bite. Chew each bite of your food at least twenty times or take 15-20 seconds to actually enjoy it.

There are numerous studies that have been conducted that reinforce our theory. In 2008, the *Journal of American Dietetic Association* published a study in which they monitored 30 women eating on two separate visits at two different rates of speed. When they ate more slowly they consumed fewer calories, drank more water, and rated their meal satisfaction higher than when they ate quickly. [4]

Another study in 2004 performed by the North American Association for the study of Obesity regulated the eating pace of subjects by utilizing beeps to delay their consumption speed. The results were similar to the previous study and they ate less food than they normally would.

Time is precious. Try and make a few simple changes in your life and take time for what is truly important. Most of our grandparents and parents worked hard to provide a better life for us than what they had, so we encourage you to leave a legacy as well. Why not teach and encourage healthy eating choices and a focus of spending quality time interacting with loved ones and others. This applies to everyone, not just parents or grandparents. You can have an influence on others regardless of what stage of life you're in. A youth can spend time with some of the older generation at church and learn a great deal. Likewise, a senior citizen can invite a young family to lunch and just spend time talking and having meaningful dialogue with them. A little bit of time spent fellowshipping with others will have more impact than if you spent four hours watching TV in silence; so spend your time wisely!

# I Can't Afford It

*I* Can't Afford It – Fast Food is so inexpensive, I can't afford to always cook.

We've been trying to encourage you to cook healthier and prepare more meals at home. Later we'll show you how to simplify your shopping as well, but in the back of your mind you might still be concerned that you can't afford to buy organic and shop each week for everything that you need. Fast food restaurants offer many of their kid's meals at an irresistible price. It seems as though you can feed your children or even yourself at a price much cheaper than you can cook. That might be true in some instances, but at what price? You're getting almost no nutritional value and you load yourself with unwanted fat calories. Price should not be the final determining factor when you or your family's health is involved. If we gave you a choice between a piece of cardboard with frosting on it or some strawberries, hopefully that would be a fairly simple decision, right? If you had to think about that for more than one second then you need to immediately put this book down and call your pastor for prayer. Cardboard with icing might look pretty and the sugar in the icing might even mask the taste of the cardboard making it palatable, but it is all deception. A colorful package, cheap price and good taste add up to absolutely nothing as far as your health is concerned. God has provided us with His own colorful packaging, inexpensive price and great taste anyway. Look at a banana and some strawberries as an example. They're the same pretty red and yellow that some fast foods try to attract you with. There are actual studies that claim the colors red and yellow increase your appetite (no wonder the three largest fast food restaurants use those colors as part of their logos). Strawberries and bananas are two of the original red and yellow color pattern designs and you can grow them for free if you have just a little bit of property. So God provided inexpensive pricing and incredible taste at his fast food restaurant.

In case you don't have the property to grow your own food or have a boat to go catch your own fresh fish, buying organic fruits and vegetables, range free eggs or wild caught fish is a little pricier, but can you truly place a price on being healthy? One of our favorite quotes comes from Leon Eldred, "If I'd known I was going to live so long, I'd have taken better care of myself." If you choose not to buy organic then take a moment and imagine what the chemicals and pesticides used on most produce are doing to your body? We're told that they use them to kill the insects and vermin, but it won't harm us. Yeah, right. So just a little cyanide won't kill me but how sick will it make me after repeated use?

If money is tight, and it is for almost all of us, then we have a simple task for you. The next time you go to the grocery store, take a pad of paper and write down the price difference between regular and organic. You might be surprised to find out that it only costs you an additional $20 per week to buy organic. So you'll need to trim $20 from your budget. That can be pretty easy to do. Increase the deductible on your car insurance, or pay off your credit card because the interest is probably costing you more than that, or fast for one meal each week and you just made up the difference.

Do you remember the last time that you had the flu or a sickness that kept you flat on your back in your bed? You were so miserable that you might have even asked the Lord, "If it's my time then just take me now!" That's a possible consequence of eating foods that are treated with chemicals to make them bigger, brighter, or more appealing. Eating organic isn't the cure-all for sickness but if it can help prevent just even one sick day per year, then isn't it worth it? Just ask any employer how much of a cost lost they experience from absenteeism due to illnesses. Consider yourself the employer of your own body. You want your staff to be as healthy and productive as possible, so plant the best seed that you can so your workforce (your own body) is healthy and invigorated to carry out the days duties. If you shop for someone other than yourself, let's say a spouse and children, now you're running an entire little corporation that you want to keep healthy. Think back on the last time you had to stay home with a sick child, how helpless you felt that as the parent that you couldn't make them feel better immediately. You wished that you could just give them a kiss on their forehead and everything would immediately be fine. That's the same way that our heavenly Father looks at us, His children. He wants us to be as healthy as possible so that we can carry out His will in our lives, but we load our bodies with garbage and then suffer the consequences. He wants to just reach down and kiss our foreheads and instantly heal us, which He sometimes does when we cry out to Him, but He has also given us free will and we often abuse that privilege. It's no different than one of our own children sneaking a bag of candy and eating so much that they make themselves sick. Buying organic produce, range and cage free eggs and poultry, and wild caught fish is a little more expensive, but what cost are you paying in the long term by dumping chemicals into your field? What will your harvest be after weeks, months or years of exposing your body to those toxins?

Who knows? If you are able to encourage all of your church and family members to start buying organic, demand will increase so additional farmers might be encouraged to switch to organic to meet the demand which will in turn eventually bring prices down because of the volume of product now produced to meet the demand. The economics of supply and demand will balance out the pricing and healthier products will become the norm. Try organic for just one month and see if it makes a difference in how you feel? If you couple that with your pledge to be more conscientious of what seed you're planting in your field, you might be surprised at how much more energy you have and how great you feel when you wake up. Planting good seed for an entire month will yield a healthy harvest where you'll feel stronger, brighter, more alert, and more productive. The sugar hangovers and lethargy from fat consumption will be symptoms of the past.

# Sin (you might want to skip this chapter)

*S*in – I know I shouldn't eat it, but a few bites won't hurt me.

*Don't read this chapter!*

Okay, you were warned. Now you have no excuse so don't email or write us a letter trying to justify your position or argue that being unhealthy can be traced to certain biblical principles, because the Bible considers overeating to be a sin. Ouch. Yes, we said it. Gluttony is a sin.

Our bodies house the Holy Spirit and therefore we are the Temple of the Holy Spirit. Because of that we are to keep them pure, free from immorality and clean. That isn't our opinion that is straight from the word of God.

> Or do you not know that your body is a temple of the Holy Spirit who is in you, whom you have from God, and that you are not your own?
>
> 1 Corinthians 6:19 (NASB)

> For the heavy drinker and the glutton will
> come to poverty, And drowsiness will clothe
> one with rags.
>
> Proverbs 23:21 (NASB)

God created you in His image. Are you honoring Him by taking care of His gift? You don't need to become obsessed and work out for 6 hours each day, just respect the precious gift that was given you. If you do work out for several hours each day or you're a body builder, we think that's fantastic as long as it doesn't become a fixation of vanity but instead you do it to glorify the Lord. There are several ways to honor your temple and utilize the resources that He has given us, including your intellect to educate yourself in making healthy decisions and taking care of yourself. The majority of prayer requests that pastors and call-in prayer lines receive are for health-related issues. God wants us to be as healthy as we can so that we can carry out His plan for our life and be a witness to others.

> And He said to them, "Go into all the world
> and preach the gospel to every creature."
>
> Mark 16:15 (NKJV)

The better health that you're in, the more effective you can be in carrying out this commission and the plans He has for you. If you say that you're a Christian, then you are a little Christ. An anointed one. You should represent Him in everything that you do. From how you treat others to every action in your daily walk. If you are unhealthy by choice, and being a glutton is a choice, then you are dishonoring your Creator. By the way, you were warned not to read this section so take a deep breath and recite the pledge from earlier that *you will start sowing the right seed for a healthy harvest*!

If you are currently living an unhealthy life, then what seeds are you sowing for your family and loved ones? Are you setting a good example for them? This isn't meant to condemn you because we're going to close this chapter with some great news. God loves you, and all you have to do is ask for His help. We have a loving heavenly Father and He is always faithful to help us. If you have asked Him to rescue you and you have turned away from sin, then you've repented. Now you can start from this day forward as a new creation and start a walk of health for you, your family, and your Heavenly Father. From this day forward you're going to be an awesome witness for Christ and have an incredible testimony of victory to share with everyone!

# Tools to Victory-Calorie Counting

We went into extensive detail in the first half of the book to outline many of the areas in your healthy journey that might cause you to stumble and hopefully we've helped you to recognize them now before you trip over them. Knowing where and when you might falter is only half of the battle. The real key to victory is having the tools to stay on track and one of the most important tools is to understand how much seed you're putting into your field. A farmer can count how many seeds he plants or measure the amount of seed that he will sow into a certain row. Since you are now the farmer of your own body you can do exactly the same thing by calorie counting. Don't get overwhelmed because this is possibly the second most important section in this book, running just slightly behind controlling your portion sizes. Counting your calories is paramount to taking charge and remaining in control of your health. This is what will help you to change and adopt a healthy lifestyle for the remainder of your life and prevent the yo-yo effect that most people experience from diets. Don't get discouraged and think that calorie counting is too much work, because it's actually very simple. How many items do you normally purchase each week at the grocery store: 40, maybe 100, possibly even 200? Pick one item to study each day, and in one year you would have 365 different food items that you are familiar with. It only takes about 5 minutes to research the calorie count on one item and that's an incredible investment of time that will pay off for the rest of your life.

Let's take one simple item; rolls. Research a few different brand names and types and you'll gain an enormous amount of knowledge about that one food. There can be a vast difference in calories depending on which type you purchase, so research several of them and learn which one would be best for you to place into your shopping cart.

1 whole wheat potato roll = 60 calories per roll.

1 whole wheat Kaiser roll made by a well known manufacturer = 200 calories per roll.

In just that one item there can be more than three times as many calories. Imagine if you made the wrong decision for each item in your meal. You could go from a very healthy 600 calorie lunch to a large 2,000 calorie time bomb by making a few simple mistakes.

Write down all of the foods for every meal that you eat for just one week and research each item so that you can start making knowledgeable, well informed decisions. It's also a great exercise at the grocery store. Grab several different packages of rolls by different manufacturers and compare their ingredients, calories and carbohydrates. You can also make a game out of it with your children. Challenge them to find the popcorn with the least amount of calories and now you'll have an entire team of food researchers working for you.

You can also start a discussion with different groups at church. Encourage everyone to share some of their own research while you contribute what you've learned about rolls or popcorn. It makes a much better topic of conversation than many other things that can creep into the church; like gossip. This would make a great way for you to steer an unpleasant conversation into something more useful by changing the subject and talking about the varying calorie counts that your kids found in popcorn.

The best thing about calorie counting is that in a few simple weeks you will already have enough education to dramatically impact your meals, and in a few months you can be an amateur nutritionist for your family.

# Calorie Deficit

*N*ow that you have a basic understanding of how important counting calories is it will make it much easier for you to create a calorie deficit. In order to lose weight, you have to create a calorie deficit, which in simple terms means to burn more calories than you take in. If you eat 2,000 calories each day, then to lose weight you need to burn more than 2,000 calories. Seems pretty basic right? Well it honestly is that simple. Don't look at 2,000 calories and get overwhelmed thinking that you could never exercise enough to burn that many calories, because we have great news for you. You will burn almost that many calories by doing nothing but breathing. A 160 pound person will burn about 550 calories while sleeping for eight hours. Then they can burn another 1,382 calories by just sitting still for 16 more hours. So by doing absolutely nothing for 24 hours, a 160 pound person will burn around 1,932 calories. Now if this same 160 pound person goes for a brisk 30-minute walk, they'll burn an additional 172 calories (550+1,382+172=2,104). So if you start with the 2,000 calories that they consumed today, and subtract the 2,104 calories that they burned today, then they have a 104 calorie deficit for the day. But if they didn't work out that day, then you need to subtract the 172 calories that they burned during their walk (2,104 − 172 = 1,932) so they now have a surplus of 68 calories (2,000 from food − 1,932 burned for the day) that they haven't burned off. Those 68 calories are now running around the body looking for a place to rest, and that place of rest might be around their waist or in their thighs. To put it in perspective, a 115 pound person will burn 1,388 calories each day by just breathing, but if they stopped and had a fast food cheeseburger, large fries and a large soda, that's 1,520 calories and no nutritional value. So they are still hungry because their body is craving some nutrition but they're already 134 calories over for the day. Do that every day and you gained 14 pounds that year by only eating one meal per day. This isn't meant to discourage you; we want to encourage you to make healthier choices by opening your eyes to the perils of fast food and the detriment of ignoring your calorie count.

Is creating a deficit of 104 calories per day a good target? Will that minor amount add up to any benefit? It depends on your goal. Here is a simple formula to see how your weight loss is progressing. One pound of body weight equals about 3,500 calories. So if you were able to stay consistent with your 104 calorie deficit each day, then it would take you 34 days (34 x 104 = 3,536) to lose one pound. If your goal is to lose 12 pounds this year, then 104 calories per day would do it. If your goal is more aggressive than that, then use this worksheet to figure out how many calories you need to burn to reach your goal. This list is based on a yearly goal because in order to live a healthier life it has to be a complete lifestyle change not just a short term goal for the upcoming wedding photos. Remember that this is for your life, not a quick fix 30 or 90 day super pill. You can starve yourself for the upcoming class reunion but you'll end up putting on more weight in the months after it's over. A sprinter going at full speed can only keep that pace up for a short distance and then they have to stop. Life isn't a sprint, it's a marathon. It's about being *consistent*. A successful farmer is *consistent* and diligent in their goal of yielding a good harvest each season. It's great to have 30, 60 and 90 day goals, which you should, but it's just as important to have a *consistent* 2, 5 and 10 year goal. A good measure of success is *consistency*. Did we mention how important *consistency* is yet? An athlete can have one spectacular game or event (which can be represented by the 10 pounds that you lost before the reunion), but in order to have a career an athlete needs to be consistent over a long period of time. Who was the winner of Wimbledon in 1980? You probably have no idea but that is an incredible accomplishment. Compare that to the consistent accomplishments of Chris Evert or Martina Navratilova. Don't let your health goals be a one time victory. Set your sight on long range goals. By the way, Evonne Goolagong Cawley defeated Chris Evert in the 1980 final of Wimbledon. Chris Evert defeated the 1979 defending champion Martina Navratilova in the semifinals before eventually losing to Cawley in the final.

You lost 10 pounds 5 years ago, three pounds the following year, and another 10 pounds over the last 3 years. Add up those five years and you are now 25 pounds lighter and living and enjoying a stronger, younger feeling and healthier life. That's the victory that you need to keep in focus, not that you lost 10 pounds back in 2005 but now you're 25 pounds heavier than you were. Set long range goals and then develop short term goals that will help you achieve the long range. One pound a month over five years is 60 pounds! At that consistent pace you might be able to get into your wedding or prom dress again. Not that you would really ever want to wear them, but just seeing yourself as your younger you is an incredible victory so be consistent and make lifestyle changes.

Daily Calorie Deficit Plan

| | example | your #'s |
|---|---|---|
| weight loss goal this year | 24lbs | lbs. |
| calories per pound | 3,500 | 3,500 |
| | (3,500 x 24) | (3,500 x      your goal in lbs.) |
| TOTAL CALORIES this year | 84,000 | total |
| | divide by 52 | divided by 52 |
| Weekly Total | 1,615 | weekly total |
| | divide by 7 | div by 7 |
| Daily Total | 230 calories | total calories per day |

This next graph will help you to determine how many calories you burn each day for almost any activity. Add your weight, how long you participated in that event, and then figure out your total calories burned during that event.

## Calories Burned Activity Chart
### How Many Calories Did You Burn?

Perform this calculation to determine how many calories your activity burned.
Activity Per Minute # x Your Body Weight x # of Minutes You Participated = Total Calories Burned

Example - You weigh 160 pounds and raked leaves in the yard for 30 minutes.
.030256 (Raking yard) x 160 (lbs.) x 30 (minutes) = 145 calories

Or find an activity below then find the column closest to your body weight and see how many calories you would burn in one hour.

(The calculations used in creating this chart were taken from the Department of Health and Family Services State of Wisconsin, Division of Public Health, PPH 40109 (06/09) )
http://www.dhs.wisconsin.gov/health/physicalactivity/pdf_files/caloriesperhour.pdf

| Activity | calories burned per hour per pound | calories burned per minute per pound | 130 lbs | 150 lbs | 180 lbs | 200 lbs | 220 lbs |
|---|---|---|---|---|---|---|---|
| Aerobics, high impact | 3.1769 | 0.052949 | 413 | 477 | 572 | 635 | 699 |
| Aerobics, low impact | 2.2692 | 0.037821 | 295 | 340 | 408 | 454 | 499 |
| Archery (nonhunting) | 1.5923 | 0.026538 | 207 | 239 | 287 | 318 | 350 |
| Automobile repair | 1.3615 | 0.022692 | 177 | 204 | 245 | 272 | 300 |
| Backpacking, general | 3.1769 | 0.052949 | 413 | 477 | 572 | 635 | 699 |
| Badminton, competitive | 3.1769 | 0.052949 | 413 | 477 | 572 | 635 | 699 |
| Badminton, social, general | 2.0462 | 0.034103 | 266 | 307 | 368 | 409 | 450 |
| Basketball, game | 3.6308 | 0.060513 | 472 | 545 | 654 | 726 | 799 |
| Basketball, nongame, general | 2.7231 | 0.045385 | 354 | 408 | 490 | 545 | 599 |
| Basketball, officiating | 3.1769 | 0.052949 | 413 | 477 | 572 | 635 | 699 |
| Basketball, shooting baskets | 2.0462 | 0.034103 | 266 | 307 | 368 | 409 | 450 |
| Basketball, wheelchair | 2.9538 | 0.049231 | 384 | 443 | 532 | 591 | 650 |
| Bicycling, <10mph, leisure | 1.8154 | 0.030256 | 236 | 272 | 327 | 363 | 399 |
| Bicycling, >20mph, racing | 7.2615 | 0.121026 | 944 | 1089 | 1307 | 1452 | 1598 |
| Bicycling, 10-11.9mph, light effort | 2.7231 | 0.045385 | 354 | 408 | 490 | 545 | 599 |
| Bicycling, 12-13.9mph, moderate effort | 3.6308 | 0.060513 | 472 | 545 | 654 | 726 | 799 |
| Bicycling, 14-15.9mph, vigorous effort | 4.5385 | 0.075641 | 590 | 681 | 817 | 908 | 998 |
| Bicycling, 16-19mph, very fast, racing | 5.4462 | 0.090769 | 708 | 817 | 980 | 1089 | 1198 |
| Bicycling, BMX or mountain | 3.8615 | 0.064359 | 502 | 579 | 695 | 772 | 850 |
| Bicycling, stationary, general | 2.2692 | 0.037821 | 295 | 340 | 408 | 454 | 499 |
| Bicycling, stationary, light effort | 2.5000 | 0.041667 | 325 | 375 | 450 | 500 | 550 |

| Activity | calories burned per hour per pound | calories burned per minute per pound | 130 lbs | 150 lbs | 180 lbs | 200 lbs | 220 lbs |
|---|---|---|---|---|---|---|---|
| Bicycling, stationary, moderate effort | 3.1769 | 0.052949 | 413 | 477 | 572 | 635 | 699 |
| Bicycling, stationary, very light effort | 1.3615 | 0.022692 | 177 | 204 | 245 | 272 | 300 |
| Bicycling, stationary, very vigorous effort | 5.6769 | 0.094615 | 738 | 852 | 1022 | 1135 | 1249 |
| Bicycling, stationary, vigorous effort | 4.7692 | 0.079487 | 620 | 715 | 858 | 954 | 1049 |
| Billiards | 1.1385 | 0.018974 | 148 | 171 | 205 | 228 | 250 |
| Bowling | 1.3615 | 0.022692 | 177 | 204 | 245 | 272 | 300 |
| Boxing, in ring, general | 5.4462 | 0.090769 | 708 | 817 | 980 | 1089 | 1198 |
| Boxing, punching bag | 2.7231 | 0.045385 | 354 | 408 | 490 | 545 | 599 |
| Boxing, sparring | 4.0846 | 0.068077 | 531 | 613 | 735 | 817 | 899 |
| Broomball | 3.1769 | 0.052949 | 413 | 477 | 572 | 635 | 699 |
| Calisthenics (pushups, sit-ups), vigorous effort | 3.6308 | 0.060513 | 472 | 545 | 654 | 726 | 799 |
| Calisthenics, home, light/moderate effort | 2.0462 | 0.034103 | 266 | 307 | 368 | 409 | 450 |
| Canoeing, on camping trip | 1.8154 | 0.030256 | 236 | 272 | 327 | 363 | 399 |
| Canoeing, rowing, >6 mph, vigorous effort | 5.4462 | 0.090769 | 708 | 817 | 980 | 1089 | 1198 |
| Canoeing, rowing, crewing, competition | 5.4462 | 0.090769 | 708 | 817 | 980 | 1089 | 1198 |
| Canoeing, rowing, light effort | 1.3615 | 0.022692 | 177 | 204 | 245 | 272 | 300 |
| Canoeing, rowing, moderate effort | 3.1769 | 0.052949 | 413 | 477 | 572 | 635 | 699 |
| Carpentry, general | 1.5923 | 0.026538 | 207 | 239 | 287 | 318 | 350 |
| Carrying heavy loads, such as bricks | 3.6308 | 0.060513 | 472 | 545 | 654 | 726 | 799 |
| Child care: sitting/kneeling-dressing, feeding | 1.3615 | 0.022692 | 177 | 204 | 245 | 272 | 300 |
| Child care: standing-dressing, feeding | 1.5923 | 0.026538 | 207 | 239 | 287 | 318 | 350 |
| Circuit training, general | 3.6308 | 0.060513 | 472 | 545 | 654 | 726 | 799 |
| Cleaning, heavy, vigorous effort | 2.0462 | 0.034103 | 266 | 307 | 368 | 409 | 450 |
| Cleaning, house, general | 1.5923 | 0.026538 | 207 | 239 | 287 | 318 | 350 |
| Cleaning, light, moderate effort | 1.1385 | 0.018974 | 148 | 171 | 205 | 228 | 250 |
| Coaching: football, soccer, basketball, etc. | 1.8154 | 0.030256 | 236 | 272 | 327 | 363 | 399 |
| Construction, outside, remodeling | 2.5000 | 0.041667 | 325 | 375 | 450 | 500 | 550 |
| Cooking or food preparation | 1.1385 | 0.018974 | 148 | 171 | 205 | 228 | 250 |
| Cricket (batting, bowling) | 2.2692 | 0.037821 | 295 | 340 | 408 | 454 | 499 |
| Croquet | 1.1385 | 0.018974 | 148 | 171 | 205 | 228 | 250 |
| Curling | 1.8154 | 0.030256 | 236 | 272 | 327 | 363 | 399 |
| Dancing, aerobic, ballet or modern, twist | 2.7231 | 0.045385 | 354 | 408 | 490 | 545 | 599 |
| Dancing, ballroom, fast | 2.5000 | 0.041667 | 325 | 375 | 450 | 500 | 550 |
| Dancing, ballroom, slow | 1.3615 | 0.022692 | 177 | 204 | 245 | 272 | 300 |
| Dancing, general | 2.0462 | 0.034103 | 266 | 307 | 368 | 409 | 450 |
| Darts, wall or lawn | 1.1385 | 0.018974 | 148 | 171 | 205 | 228 | 250 |
| Diving, springboard or platform | 1.3615 | 0.022692 | 177 | 204 | 245 | 272 | 300 |
| Electrical work, plumbing | 1.5923 | 0.026538 | 207 | 239 | 287 | 318 | 350 |
| Farming, baling hay, cleaning barn | 3.6308 | 0.060513 | 472 | 545 | 654 | 726 | 799 |
| Farming, milking by hand | 1.3615 | 0.022692 | 177 | 204 | 245 | 272 | 300 |
| Farming, shoveling grain | 2.5000 | 0.041667 | 325 | 375 | 450 | 500 | 550 |
| Fencing | 2.7231 | 0.045385 | 354 | 408 | 490 | 545 | 599 |
| Fishing from boat, sitting | 1.1385 | 0.018974 | 148 | 171 | 205 | 228 | 250 |
| Fishing from river bank, standing | 1.5923 | 0.026538 | 207 | 239 | 287 | 318 | 350 |
| Fishing in stream, in waders | 2.7231 | 0.045385 | 354 | 408 | 490 | 545 | 599 |
| Fishing, general | 1.8154 | 0.030256 | 236 | 272 | 327 | 363 | 399 |
| Fishing, ice, sitting | 0.9077 | 0.015128 | 118 | 136 | 163 | 182 | 200 |
| Football or baseball, playing catch | 1.1385 | 0.018974 | 148 | 171 | 205 | 228 | 250 |
| Football, competitive | 4.0846 | 0.068077 | 531 | 613 | 735 | 817 | 899 |
| Football, touch, flag, general | 3.6308 | 0.060513 | 472 | 545 | 654 | 726 | 799 |
| Frisbee playing, general | 1.3615 | 0.022692 | 177 | 204 | 245 | 272 | 300 |
| Frisbee, ultimate | 1.5923 | 0.026538 | 207 | 239 | 287 | 318 | 350 |
| Gardening, general | 2.2692 | 0.037821 | 295 | 340 | 408 | 454 | 499 |
| Golf, carrying clubs | 2.5000 | 0.041667 | 325 | 375 | 450 | 500 | 550 |
| Golf, general | 1.8154 | 0.030256 | 236 | 272 | 327 | 363 | 399 |
| Golf, miniature or driving range | 1.3615 | 0.022692 | 177 | 204 | 245 | 272 | 300 |
| Golf, pulling clubs | 2.2692 | 0.037821 | 295 | 340 | 408 | 454 | 499 |

| Activity | calories burned per hour per pound | calories burned per minute per pound | 130 lbs | 150 lbs | 180 lbs | 200 lbs | 220 lbs |
|---|---|---|---|---|---|---|---|
| Golf, using power cart | 1.5923 | 0.026538 | 207 | 239 | 287 | 318 | 350 |
| Gymnastics, general | 1.8154 | 0.030256 | 236 | 272 | 327 | 363 | 399 |
| Hacky sack | 1.8154 | 0.030256 | 236 | 272 | 327 | 363 | 399 |
| Handball, general | 5.4462 | 0.090769 | 708 | 817 | 980 | 1089 | 1198 |
| Handball, team | 3.6308 | 0.060513 | 472 | 545 | 654 | 726 | 799 |
| Health club exercise, general | 2.5000 | 0.041667 | 325 | 375 | 450 | 500 | 550 |
| Hiking, cross country | 2.7231 | 0.045385 | 354 | 408 | 490 | 545 | 599 |
| Hockey, field | 3.6308 | 0.060513 | 472 | 545 | 654 | 726 | 799 |
| Hockey, ice | 3.6308 | 0.060513 | 472 | 545 | 654 | 726 | 799 |
| Horse grooming | 2.7231 | 0.045385 | 354 | 408 | 490 | 545 | 599 |
| Horse racing, galloping | 3.6308 | 0.060513 | 472 | 545 | 654 | 726 | 799 |
| Horseback riding, general | 1.8154 | 0.030256 | 236 | 272 | 327 | 363 | 399 |
| Horseback riding, trotting | 2.9538 | 0.049231 | 384 | 443 | 532 | 591 | 650 |
| Horseback riding, walking | 1.1385 | 0.018974 | 148 | 171 | 205 | 228 | 250 |
| Hunting, general | 2.2692 | 0.037821 | 295 | 340 | 408 | 454 | 499 |
| Jai alai | 5.4462 | 0.090769 | 708 | 817 | 980 | 1089 | 1198 |
| Jogging, general | 3.1769 | 0.052949 | 413 | 477 | 572 | 635 | 699 |
| Judo, karate, kick boxing, tae kwan do | 4.5385 | 0.075641 | 590 | 681 | 817 | 908 | 998 |
| Kayaking | 2.2692 | 0.037821 | 295 | 340 | 408 | 454 | 499 |
| Kickball | 3.1769 | 0.052949 | 413 | 477 | 572 | 635 | 699 |
| Lacrosse | 3.6308 | 0.060513 | 472 | 545 | 654 | 726 | 799 |
| Marching band, playing instrument(walking) | 1.8154 | 0.030256 | 236 | 272 | 327 | 363 | 399 |
| Marching, rapidly, military | 2.9538 | 0.049231 | 384 | 443 | 532 | 591 | 650 |
| Moto-cross | 1.8154 | 0.030256 | 236 | 272 | 327 | 363 | 399 |
| Moving furniture, household | 2.7231 | 0.045385 | 354 | 408 | 490 | 545 | 599 |
| Moving household items, boxes, upstairs | 4.0846 | 0.068077 | 531 | 613 | 735 | 817 | 899 |
| Moving household items, carrying boxes | 3.1769 | 0.052949 | 413 | 477 | 572 | 635 | 699 |
| Mowing lawn, general | 2.5000 | 0.041667 | 325 | 375 | 450 | 500 | 550 |
| Mowing lawn, riding mower | 1.1385 | 0.018974 | 148 | 171 | 205 | 228 | 250 |
| Music playing, cello, flute, horn, woodwind | 0.9077 | 0.015128 | 118 | 136 | 163 | 182 | 200 |
| Music playing, drums | 1.8154 | 0.030256 | 236 | 272 | 327 | 363 | 399 |
| Music playing, guitar, classical, folk(sitting) | 0.9077 | 0.015128 | 118 | 136 | 163 | 182 | 200 |
| Music playing, guitar, rock/roll band(standing) | 1.3615 | 0.022692 | 177 | 204 | 245 | 272 | 300 |
| Music playing, piano, organ, violin, trumpet | 1.1385 | 0.018974 | 148 | 171 | 205 | 228 | 250 |
| Paddleboat | 1.8154 | 0.030256 | 236 | 272 | 327 | 363 | 399 |
| Painting, papering, plastering, scraping | 2.0462 | 0.034103 | 266 | 307 | 368 | 409 | 450 |
| Polo | 3.6308 | 0.060513 | 472 | 545 | 654 | 726 | 799 |
| Pushing or pulling stroller with child | 1.1385 | 0.018974 | 148 | 171 | 205 | 228 | 250 |
| Race walking | 2.9538 | 0.049231 | 384 | 443 | 532 | 591 | 650 |
| Racquetball, casual, general | 3.1769 | 0.052949 | 413 | 477 | 572 | 635 | 699 |
| Racquetball, competitive | 4.5385 | 0.075641 | 590 | 681 | 817 | 908 | 998 |
| Raking lawn | 1.8154 | 0.030256 | 236 | 272 | 327 | 363 | 399 |
| Rock climbing, ascending rock | 4.9923 | 0.083205 | 649 | 749 | 899 | 998 | 1098 |
| Rock climbing, rapelling | 3.6308 | 0.060513 | 472 | 545 | 654 | 726 | 799 |
| Rope jumping, fast | 5.4462 | 0.090769 | 708 | 817 | 980 | 1089 | 1198 |
| Rope jumping, moderate, general | 4.5385 | 0.075641 | 590 | 681 | 817 | 908 | 998 |
| Rope jumping, slow | 3.6308 | 0.060513 | 472 | 545 | 654 | 726 | 799 |
| Rowing, stationary, light effort | 4.3154 | 0.071923 | 561 | 647 | 777 | 863 | 949 |
| Rowing, stationary, moderate effort | 3.1769 | 0.052949 | 413 | 477 | 572 | 635 | 699 |
| Rowing, stationary, very vigorous effort | 5.4462 | 0.090769 | 708 | 817 | 980 | 1089 | 1198 |
| Rowing, stationary, vigorous effort | 3.8615 | 0.064359 | 502 | 579 | 695 | 772 | 850 |
| Rugby | 4.5385 | 0.075641 | 590 | 681 | 817 | 908 | 998 |
| Running, 10 mph (6 min mile) | 7.2615 | 0.121026 | 944 | 1089 | 1307 | 1452 | 1598 |
| Running, 10.9 mph (5.5 min mile) | 8.1692 | 0.136154 | 1062 | 1225 | 1470 | 1634 | 1797 |
| Running, 5 mph (12 min mile) | 3.6308 | 0.060513 | 472 | 545 | 654 | 726 | 799 |

| Activity | calories burned per hour per pound | calories burned per minute per pound | 130 lbs | 150 lbs | 180 lbs | 200 lbs | 220 lbs |
|---|---|---|---|---|---|---|---|
| Running, 5.2 mph (11.5 min mile) | 4.0846 | 0.068077 | 531 | 613 | 735 | 817 | 899 |
| Running, 6 mph (10 min mile) | 4.5385 | 0.075641 | 590 | 681 | 817 | 908 | 998 |
| Running, 6.7 mph (9 min mile) | 4.9923 | 0.083205 | 649 | 749 | 899 | 998 | 1098 |
| Running, 7 mph (8.5 min mile) | 5.2231 | 0.087051 | 679 | 783 | 940 | 1045 | 1149 |
| Running, 7.5mph (8 min mile) | 5.6769 | 0.094615 | 738 | 852 | 1022 | 1135 | 1249 |
| Running, 8 mph (7.5 min mile) | 6.1308 | 0.102179 | 797 | 920 | 1104 | 1226 | 1349 |
| Running, 8.6 mph (7 min mile) | 6.3538 | 0.105897 | 826 | 953 | 1144 | 1271 | 1398 |
| Running, 9 mph (6.5 min mile) | 6.8077 | 0.113462 | 885 | 1021 | 1225 | 1362 | 1498 |
| Running, cross country | 4.0846 | 0.068077 | 531 | 613 | 735 | 817 | 899 |
| Running, general | 3.6308 | 0.060513 | 472 | 545 | 654 | 726 | 799 |
| Running, in place | 3.6308 | 0.060513 | 472 | 545 | 654 | 726 | 799 |
| Running, on a track, team practice | 4.5385 | 0.075641 | 590 | 681 | 817 | 908 | 998 |
| Running, stairs, up | 6.8077 | 0.113462 | 885 | 1021 | 1225 | 1362 | 1498 |
| Running, training, pushing wheelchair | 3.6308 | 0.060513 | 472 | 545 | 654 | 726 | 799 |
| Running, wheeling, general | 1.3615 | 0.022692 | 177 | 204 | 245 | 272 | 300 |
| Sailing, boat/board, windsurfing, general | 1.3615 | 0.022692 | 177 | 204 | 245 | 272 | 300 |
| Sailing, in competition | 2.2692 | 0.037821 | 295 | 340 | 408 | 454 | 499 |
| Scrubbing floors, on hands and knees | 2.5000 | 0.041667 | 325 | 375 | 450 | 500 | 550 |
| Shoveling snow, by hand | 2.7231 | 0.045385 | 354 | 408 | 490 | 545 | 599 |
| Shuffleboard, lawn bowling | 1.3615 | 0.022692 | 177 | 204 | 245 | 272 | 300 |
| Sitting-playing with children-light | 1.1385 | 0.018974 | 148 | 171 | 205 | 228 | 250 |
| Skateboarding | 2.2692 | 0.037821 | 295 | 340 | 408 | 454 | 499 |
| Skating, ice, 9 mph or less | 2.5000 | 0.041667 | 325 | 375 | 450 | 500 | 550 |
| Skating, ice, general | 3.1769 | 0.052949 | 413 | 477 | 572 | 635 | 699 |
| Skating, ice, rapidly, > 9 mph | 4.0846 | 0.068077 | 531 | 613 | 735 | 817 | 899 |
| Skating, ice, speed, competitive | 6.8077 | 0.113462 | 885 | 1021 | 1225 | 1362 | 1498 |
| Skating, roller | 3.1769 | 0.052949 | 413 | 477 | 572 | 635 | 699 |
| Ski jumping (climb up carrying skis) | 3.1769 | 0.052949 | 413 | 477 | 572 | 635 | 699 |
| Ski machine, general | 4.3154 | 0.071923 | 561 | 647 | 777 | 863 | 949 |
| Skiing, cross-country, >8.0 mph, racing | 6.3538 | 0.105897 | 826 | 953 | 1144 | 1271 | 1398 |
| Skiing, cross-country, moderate effort | 3.6308 | 0.060513 | 472 | 545 | 654 | 726 | 799 |
| Skiing, cross-country, slow or light effort | 3.1769 | 0.052949 | 413 | 477 | 572 | 635 | 699 |
| Skiing, cross-country, uphill, maximum effort | 7.4923 | 0.124872 | 974 | 1124 | 1349 | 1498 | 1648 |
| Skiing, cross-country, vigorous effort | 4.0846 | 0.068077 | 531 | 613 | 735 | 817 | 899 |
| Skiing, downhill, light effort | 2.2692 | 0.037821 | 295 | 340 | 408 | 454 | 499 |
| Skiing, downhill, moderate effort | 2.7231 | 0.045385 | 354 | 408 | 490 | 545 | 599 |
| Skiing, downhill, vigorous effort, racing | 3.6308 | 0.060513 | 472 | 545 | 654 | 726 | 799 |
| Skiing, snow, general | 3.1769 | 0.052949 | 413 | 477 | 572 | 635 | 699 |
| Skiing, water | 2.7231 | 0.045385 | 354 | 408 | 490 | 545 | 599 |
| Ski-mobiling, water | 3.1769 | 0.052949 | 413 | 477 | 572 | 635 | 699 |
| Skin diving, scuba diving, general | 3.1769 | 0.052949 | 413 | 477 | 572 | 635 | 699 |
| Sledding, tobogganing, bobsledding, luge | 3.1769 | 0.052949 | 413 | 477 | 572 | 635 | 699 |
| Snorkeling | 2.2692 | 0.037821 | 295 | 340 | 408 | 454 | 499 |
| Snow shoeing | 3.6308 | 0.060513 | 472 | 545 | 654 | 726 | 799 |
| Snowmobiling | 1.5923 | 0.026538 | 207 | 239 | 287 | 318 | 350 |
| Soccer, casual, general | 3.1769 | 0.052949 | 413 | 477 | 572 | 635 | 699 |
| Soccer, competitive | 4.5385 | 0.075641 | 590 | 681 | 817 | 908 | 998 |
| Softball or baseball, fast or slow pitch | 2.2692 | 0.037821 | 295 | 340 | 408 | 454 | 499 |
| Softball, officiating | 2.7231 | 0.045385 | 354 | 408 | 490 | 545 | 599 |
| Squash | 5.4462 | 0.090769 | 708 | 817 | 980 | 1089 | 1198 |
| Stair-treadmill ergometer, general | 2.7231 | 0.045385 | 354 | 408 | 490 | 545 | 599 |
| Standing-packing/unpacking boxes | 1.5923 | 0.026538 | 207 | 239 | 287 | 318 | 350 |
| Stretching, hatha yoga | 1.8154 | 0.030256 | 236 | 272 | 327 | 363 | 399 |
| Surfing, body or board | 1.3615 | 0.022692 | 177 | 204 | 245 | 272 | 300 |
| Sweeping garage, sidewalk | 1.8154 | 0.030256 | 236 | 272 | 327 | 363 | 399 |
| Swimming laps, freestyle, fast, vigorous effort | 4.5385 | 0.075641 | 590 | 681 | 817 | 908 | 998 |
| Swimming laps, freestyle, light/moderate effort | 3.6308 | 0.060513 | 472 | 545 | 654 | 726 | 799 |

| Activity | calories burned per hour per pound | calories burned per minute per pound | 130 lbs | 150 lbs | 180 lbs | 200 lbs | 220 lbs |
|---|---|---|---|---|---|---|---|
| Swimming, backstroke, general | 3.6308 | 0.060513 | 472 | 545 | 654 | 726 | 799 |
| Swimming, breaststroke, general | 4.5385 | 0.075641 | 590 | 681 | 817 | 908 | 998 |
| Swimming, butterfly, general | 4.9923 | 0.083205 | 649 | 749 | 899 | 998 | 1098 |
| Swimming, leisurely, general | 2.7231 | 0.045385 | 354 | 408 | 490 | 545 | 599 |
| Swimming, sidestroke, general | 3.6308 | 0.060513 | 472 | 545 | 654 | 726 | 799 |
| Swimming, sychronized | 3.6308 | 0.060513 | 472 | 545 | 654 | 726 | 799 |
| Swimming, treading water, fast/vigorous | 4.5385 | 0.075641 | 590 | 681 | 817 | 908 | 998 |
| Swimming, treading water, moderate effort | 1.8154 | 0.030256 | 236 | 272 | 327 | 363 | 399 |
| Table tennis, ping pong | 1.8154 | 0.030256 | 236 | 272 | 327 | 363 | 399 |
| Tai chi | 1.8154 | 0.030256 | 236 | 272 | 327 | 363 | 399 |
| Teaching aerobics class | 2.7231 | 0.045385 | 354 | 408 | 490 | 545 | 599 |
| Tennis, doubles | 2.7231 | 0.045385 | 354 | 408 | 490 | 545 | 599 |
| Tennis, general | 3.1769 | 0.052949 | 413 | 477 | 572 | 635 | 699 |
| Tennis, singles | 3.6308 | 0.060513 | 472 | 545 | 654 | 726 | 799 |
| Unicycling | 2.2692 | 0.037821 | 295 | 340 | 408 | 454 | 499 |
| Volleyball, beach | 3.6308 | 0.060513 | 472 | 545 | 654 | 726 | 799 |
| Volleyball, competitive, in gymnasium | 1.8154 | 0.030256 | 236 | 272 | 327 | 363 | 399 |
| Volleyball, noncompetitive; 6-9 member team | 1.3615 | 0.022692 | 177 | 204 | 245 | 272 | 300 |
| Walk/run-playing with children-moderate | 1.8154 | 0.030256 | 236 | 272 | 327 | 363 | 399 |
| Walk/run-playing with children-vigorous | 2.2692 | 0.037821 | 295 | 340 | 408 | 454 | 499 |
| Walking, 2.0 mph, slow pace | 1.1385 | 0.018974 | 148 | 171 | 205 | 228 | 250 |
| Walking, 3.0 mph, mod. pace, walking dog | 1.5923 | 0.026538 | 207 | 239 | 287 | 318 | 350 |
| Walking, 3.5 mph, uphill | 2.7231 | 0.045385 | 354 | 408 | 490 | 545 | 599 |
| Walking, 4.0 mph, very brisk pace | 1.8154 | 0.030256 | 236 | 272 | 327 | 363 | 399 |
| Walking, carrying infant or 15-lb load | 1.5923 | 0.026538 | 207 | 239 | 287 | 318 | 350 |
| Walking, grass track | 2.2692 | 0.037821 | 295 | 340 | 408 | 454 | 499 |
| Walking, upstairs | 3.6308 | 0.060513 | 472 | 545 | 654 | 726 | 799 |
| Walking, using crutches | 1.8154 | 0.030256 | 236 | 272 | 327 | 363 | 399 |
| Wallyball, general | 3.1769 | 0.052949 | 413 | 477 | 572 | 635 | 699 |
| Water aerobics, water calisthenics | 1.8154 | 0.030256 | 236 | 272 | 327 | 363 | 399 |
| Water polo | 4.5385 | 0.075641 | 590 | 681 | 817 | 908 | 998 |
| Water volleyball | 1.3615 | 0.022692 | 177 | 204 | 245 | 272 | 300 |
| Weight lifting or body building, vigorous effort | 2.7231 | 0.045385 | 354 | 408 | 490 | 545 | 599 |
| Weight lifting, light or moderate effort | 1.3615 | 0.022692 | 177 | 204 | 245 | 272 | 300 |
| Whitewater rafting, kayaking, or canoeing | 2.2692 | 0.037821 | 295 | 340 | 408 | 454 | 499 |

To summarize this lesson on creating a calorie deficit, we're going to oversimplify it for you. Imagine trying to force, pack or cram 400 ounces of Jell-O (which represents eating 4,000 calories that day) into a cup that only holds 200 ounces (which represents your bodies 2,000 calorie limit). You can push and squeeze as much as you want but you're going to end up with Jell-O oozing between your fingers and squirting out everywhere. That Jell-O overflow represents the extra calories that are roaming your body looking for a place to settle which can sometimes be the reason that your pants seem to have shrunk.

We do have a special note that you need to pay attention to. As you begin to lose pounds and get closer to your optimal weight, the amount of calories that you need to burn will change because your overall weight has changed. For example, if you've lost 15 pounds over the last 3 months, then your calorie deficit formula will need to be revised. You will need to consume fewer calories or increase your exercise so that you burn more calories. You can't stay on the same program that you were 15 pounds ago or you will plateau and become stagnant. You will need to make your *calorie deficit plan* a sliding scale to counteract the weight loss as you continue your journey.

The next chapter is going to outline some great news that will help you with your calorie deficit. Muscle burns more calories than fat, so if you can adopt a good resistance training program (weights, dumbbells, bands), then you will be increasing and improving your muscular structure so you will be burning more calories automatically, even when at rest. So keep reading and get ready for your blessing as you sow healthier seed.

# Muscle Burns More Calories than Fat

*N*ow that you've learned how to eat healthier we're going to show you how to increase your metabolism. People use every excuse imaginable to justify why they are unhealthy. Everything from being big boned to having a slow metabolism. As much as you may try and convince yourself that there is an outside force that is preventing you from being healthier, neither of these is a legitimate or valid excuse. The good news is that there is a solution and exercise is the final piece of the puzzle for your journey. It will actually increase the amount of calories that you burn, even while you're resting. Not only will you lose weight, you will gain strength at the same time and increase your vitality.

Muscle weighs more than fat and it also burns more calories than fat. We want to encourage you not to get too hung up on what the scale says because two people with identical weights can be on the opposite spectrum of health. Think about an NFL running back that is in incredible shape but because of the musculature of their

body they are fairly heavy at 230 pounds and only 5'11"
tall. If you just go by their height to weight ratio they
would be classified as obese. Compare that to someone
that is also 5'11" and 230 pounds but they have trouble
seeing their shoes without leaning forward. That's one
of the reasons the scale is not always the best gauge
for your progress. If you start a comprehensive exercise
program you will immediately begin to burn calories
and drop pounds at an encouraging pace; but after a few
months of staying disciplined with your workouts you
will start to add muscle which can cause frustration if
you just go by the scale. Don't let the scale be your only
measuring tool for how successful your efforts are. How
your clothes fit is a great gauge of your progress but
our favorite testament to your success is how you feel.
As you begin to sow healthier seed into your field and
exercise regularly; you will sleep better, wake up more
refreshed and feel more alert and energized throughout
the day. That is the ultimate goal and pinnacle of waving
your fat goodbye for good.

If you are currently exercising regularly or have just
begun a program, you will reach plateaus every few
weeks or months so make sure and vary your workouts
to keep your body and muscles engaged. Your exercise
program needs to incorporate a variety of different
workouts and ideally some sort of hobby along with
it so that your mind will stay as active and involved as
your body. The majority of people stop their exercise
program because of boredom so the following program
is designed to keep you motivated and involved. The
first thing that you have to do is get a partner or better

yet, an entire group involved with you. It's much easier to stay motivated if you have others depending on you and it creates accountability to keep you on track. You can find a partner or form a group at your church, at your local YMCA, or any local fitness center.

We want you to make sure that you do one thing when exercising or determining what new hobby you might pursue...*have fun*! The majority of people dread working out so that makes it pretty easy to miss a day or skip an entire week or two. Honestly, how much fun is it to sit on a stationary bike for 30 minutes, pedaling your little heart out as the sweat pools underneath you, and not actually getting anywhere? Or walking in the same spot on a treadmill (like a hamster on his wheel) and not getting even one block closer to your destination?

To increase your potential for fun and consistency try to spend a few days each week in an activity that you truly enjoy as a hobby. Perhaps join a local softball league, morning walking club, a volleyball league, golfing group, flag football, square dancing, bicycling club, soccer, badminton, lawn bowling, or start a weekly kickball game with your family and neighborhood kids. Whatever you enjoy doing, find one or two days each week to get together with your group; have fun and get active.

Once you've picked a hobby or activity, the rest of your exercise routine will now have much more meaning and focus because while you're strength training and working on your conditioning, you can relate it to your hobby. You can work on specific training areas that will make your hobby more enjoyable and increase your aptitude in it. If you're playing softball then work on your thigh strength, hip flexibility, hip rotation speed, forearm and shoulder strength, shoulder flexibility and range of motion.

Once you have a plan and purpose for resistance training (lifting weights or using machines), instead of just pushing an iron plate, you'll be able to envision the act of hitting the ball harder and driving in the winning run, or throwing someone out at first after making a back handed grab deep behind third base. Or it might be as simple as increasing your strength, cardio and coordination so that you can make the one mile walk with your grandchildren to take them to the park.

Whatever your goal is, make it fun focused so that you can stay motivated and involved.

The goal is for you to develop your own exercise plan that incorporates daily activities and a hobby to keep you healthy. To get you started here is a simple 30-day exercise plan to jumpstart your metabolism. We need you to commit just thirty minutes, 6 days a week. As recommended earlier, get a group together to help you, but all of these can be done right in your own home, so there is no excuse. If you can't find thirty minutes six days each week, then you're too busy. You need to simplify your life and set aside the things of the world for just a few minutes and focus on you and your family's health.

We're providing you with a 30-day exercise regiment that you can get the entire family involved in. It's a quick thirty minute per day program designed for anyone at any fitness level, from beginners to the advanced. We're encouraging you to commit to trying it for thirty days and we can guarantee that you will see results. Here is your thirty day list, but don't get overwhelmed, there is a beginner, intermediate and advanced level for you to follow. Since working out with a partner is so much better for you, grab some family members and make it a workout party.

# 30-Day Exercise Plan

*D*o you watch at least 30 minutes of TV each day? Then you have time to exercise. The average American watches almost 4 hours of television each day so if they would learn to exercise while watching TV then we could almost completely eliminate obesity in America. The "Wave Your Fat Goodbye" exercise routine is designed to complete in just 30 minutes and the majority of it can be done right in your own living room. The program is designed as a form of burst training where you put in 100% of your effort for a short period and then rest for a short period before pushing yourself again as hard as you can. If you had a track to run on then imagine sprinting for 60 yards, then walking for 60 yards, and then sprinting for another 60. You would repeat that cycle for 2 minutes and then take a one-minute break. This form of burst training has been proven to be extremely effective in building muscle, increasing stamina, and strengthening your heart. The "Wave Your Fat Goodbye" exercise routine also incorporates mixing up your workouts so that your body is constantly adapting, getting plenty of rest to recuperate, and increasing in flexibility and coordination.

The first week is designed to work every body part with resistance using dumbbells or some kind of weight. Push yourself as hard as you can for 15 seconds and then take a 15 second break. You'll repeat the 15 second on/off cycle for a full 2 minutes and then take a one-minute break before you start the next round. If you have a question about how to perform an exercise, visit our website for a tutorial at www.WaveYourFatGoodbye.com.

# Week one: 15second burst / :15second rest (for 2 minutes then a 1 minute break)

## Monday (weights / dumbbells) - arms & shoulders

Round 1–military press
Round 2–front raises
Round 3–lateral raises
Round 4–upright row
Round 5–overhead tricep extension
Round 6–curls
Round 7–hammer curls
Round 8–wrist curls
Round 9–repeat 4–round 2, 3, 4, 1

## Tuesday - cardio & stretching

30 minutes of cardio (walk, bike, run, punching heavy bag, swim, jump rope or aerobics)

30 minutes of stretching (can even be done while watching TV – calf, hamstring, quad, stomach, arm, shoulder, wrist, neck)

## Wednesday-(weights or bands) - legs & stomach

Round 1–dead lifts
Round 2–squats
Round 3–calf raises
Round 4–lunges
Round 5–side to side shift
Round 6–seated knee lifts
Round 7–seated leg lifts
Round 8–seated bicycle
Round 9–repeat 4–round 2, 3, 7, 6

## Thursday (weights / dumbbells) - back, chest & neck

Round 1–bench press
Round 2–alternating bench press
Round 3–incline bench
Round 4–flys
Round 5–bent over row
Round 6–lawn mower pull
Round 7–staggered push-up
Round 8–tricep push-up
Round 9–repeat 4–round 1, 4, 5, 6

## Friday - walk, hobby & stretching

30-minute walk after dinner and 30 minutes of hobby (walk / hobby – softball, golf, volleyball, tennis)

30 minutes of stretching (while you watch TV – calf, hamstring, quad, stomach, arm, shoulder, wrist, neck)

## Saturday Special - full body cardio and weights combo

2min. Exercise + 1 min. Isometric

(keep a record of the number of reps that you complete and try to improve upon it each Saturday)

Round 1–2 minutes–push ups
Round 1–1 minute isometric–horse stance
Round 2–2 minutes–squats
Round 2–1 minute isometric–jockey stance
Round 3–2 minutes–clean and press
Round 3–1 minute isometric–horse stance
Round 4–2 minutes–jumps
Round 4–1 minute isometric–jockey stance
Round 5- 2 minutes–dead lift
Round 5–1 minute isometric–horse stance
Round 6–2 minutes–jumping jacks
Round 6–1 minute isometric–jockey stance
Round 7–2 minutes–v sit-ups
Round 7–1 minute isometric–horse stance
Round 8–2 minutes–leg flutter
Round 8–1 minute isometric–jockey stance
Round 9–2 minutes–mountain climber
Round 9–1 minute isometric–horse stance

## Sunday - walk, hobby & stretching

30-minute walk after dinner and 30 minutes of hobby (walk / hobby – softball, golf, volleyball, tennis)

30 minutes of stretching (calf, hamstring, quad, stomach, arm, shoulder, wrist, neck) Week One: 15second burst / :15second rest (for 2 minutes then a 1 minute break)

## Week two - 2 minutes on / 1 minute rest (full 2 minutes to exhaustion)

The second week is designed to push your muscles to exhaustion. Complete each two minute round without stopping then take a one-minute break before the next round. Push yourself as hard as you can during the two minutes so that you are out of breath before taking the one-minute break.

### Monday (weights / dumbbells) - arms & shoulders

Round 1—military press
Round 2—front raises
Round 3—lateral raises
Round 4—upright row
Round 5—overhead tricep extension
Round 6—curls
Round 7—hammer curls
Round 8—wrist curls
Round 9—repeat 4—round 2, 3, 4, 1

### Tuesday - cardio & stretching

30 minutes of cardio (walk, bike, run, punching heavy bag, swim, jump rope or aerobics)

30 minutes of stretching (can even be done while watching TV – calf, hamstring, quad, stomach, arm, shoulder, wrist, neck)

## Wednesday-(weights or bands) - legs & stomach

Round 1–dead lifts
Round 2–squats
Round 3–calf raises
Round 4–lunges
Round 5–side to side shift
Round 6–seated knee lifts
Round 7–seated leg lifts
Round 8–seated bicycle
Round 9–repeat 4–round 2, 3, 7, 6

## Thursday (weights / dumbbells) - back, chest & neck

Round 1–bench press
Round 2–alternating bench press
Round 3–incline bench
Round 4–flys
Round 5–bent over row
Round 6–lawn mower pull
Round 7–staggered push-up
Round 8–tricep push-up
Round 9–repeat 4–round 1, 4, 5, 6

## Friday - walk, hobby & stretching

30-minute walk after dinner and 30 minutes of hobby (walk / hobby – softball, golf, volleyball, tennis)

30 minutes of stretching (while you watch TV – calf, hamstring, quad, stomach, arm, shoulder, wrist, neck)

## Saturday Special - full body cardio and weights combo

2min. Exercise + 1 min. Isometric
(keep a record of the number of reps that you complete and try to improve upon it each Saturday)
Round 1–2 minutes–push ups
Round 1–1 minute isometric–horse stance
Round 2–2 minutes–squats
Round 2–1 minute isometric–jockey stance
Round 3–2 minutes–clean and press
Round 3–1 minute isometric–horse stance
Round 4–2 minutes–jumps
Round 4–1 minute isometric–jockey stance
Round 5- 2 minutes–dead lift
Round 5–1 minute isometric–horse stance
Round 6–2 minutes–jumping jacks
Round 6–1 minute isometric–jockey stance
Round 7–2 minutes–v sit-ups
Round 7–1 minute isometric–horse stance
Round 8–2 minutes–leg flutter
Round 8–1 minute isometric–jockey stance
Round 9–2 minutes–mountain climber
Round 9–1 minute isometric–horse stance

## Sunday - walk, hobby & stretching

30-minute walk after dinner and 30 minutes of hobby (walk / hobby – softball, golf, volleyball, tennis)
30 minutes of stretching (calf, hamstring, quad, stomach, arm, shoulder, wrist, neck)

# Week three: 10 second burst / :10 second rest (for 2 minutes then a 1 minute break)

Week three is designed to build more muscle. Use heavier weights and push yourself for 10 seconds then take a 10 second break before pushing as hard as you can for another 10 seconds. Use enough weight that you don't think you could do even one more repetition at the end of 10 seconds.

## Monday (weights / dumbbells) - arms & shoulders

Round 1—military press
Round 2—front raises
Round 3—lateral raises
Round 4—upright row
Round 5—overhead tricep extension
Round 6—curls
Round 7—hammer curls
Round 8—wrist curls
Round 9—repeat 4—round 2, 3, 4, 1

## Tuesday - cardio & stretching

30 minutes of cardio (walk, bike, run, punching heavy bag, swim, jump rope or aerobics)

30 minutes of stretching (can even be done while watching TV — calf, hamstring, quad, stomach, arm, shoulder, wrist, neck)

## Wednesday-(weights or bands) - legs & stomach

Round 1—dead lifts

Round 2–squats
Round 3–calf raises
Round 4–lunges
Round 5–side to side shift
Round 6–seated knee lifts
Round 7–seated leg lifts
Round 8–seated bicycle
Round 9–repeat 4–round 2, 3, 7, 6

## Thursday (weights / dumbbells) - back, chest & neck

Round 1–bench press
Round 2–alternating bench press
Round 3–incline bench
Round 4–flys
Round 5–bent over row
Round 6–lawn mower pull
Round 7–staggered push-up
Round 8–tricep push-up
Round 9–repeat 4–round 1, 4, 5, 6

## Friday - walk, hobby & stretching

30-minute walk after dinner and 30 minutes of hobby (walk / hobby – softball, golf, volleyball, tennis)

30 minutes of stretching (while you watch TV – calf, hamstring, quad, stomach, arm, shoulder, wrist, neck)

## Saturday Special - full body cardio and weights combo

2min. Exercise + 1 min. Isometric

(keep a record of the number of reps that you complete and try to improve upon it each Saturday)

Round 1–2 minutes–push ups
Round 1–1 minute isometric–horse stance
Round 2–2 minutes–squats
Round 2–1 minute isometric–jockey stance
Round 3–2 minutes–clean and press
Round 3–1 minute isometric–horse stance
Round 4–2 minutes–jumps
Round 4–1 minute isometric–jockey stance
Round 5- 2 minutes–dead lift
Round 5–1 minute isometric–horse stance
Round 6–2 minutes–jumping jacks
Round 6–1 minute isometric–jockey stance
Round 7–2 minutes–v sit-ups
Round 7–1 minute isometric–horse stance
Round 8–2 minutes–leg flutter
Round 8–1 minute isometric–jockey stance
Round 9–2 minutes–mountain climber
Round 9–1 minute isometric–horse stance

## Sunday - walk, hobby & stretching

30-minute walk after dinner and 30 minutes of hobby (walk / hobby – softball, golf, volleyball, tennis)

30 minutes of stretching (calf, hamstring, quad, stomach, arm, shoulder, wrist, neck)

# Week four: 2 full minutes / 1 minute break

Week four is the culmination of your last three weeks and will focus on building up your stamina. Reduce the weight that you used in week three a little and push yourself through the entire two minute round.

## Monday (weights / dumbbells) - arms & shoulders

Round 1–military press
Round 2–front raises
Round 3–lateral raises
Round 4–upright row
Round 5–overhead tricep extension
Round 6–curls
Round 7–hammer curls
Round 8–wrist curls
Round 9–repeat 4–round 2, 3, 4, 1

## Tuesday - cardio & stretching

30 minutes of cardio (walk, bike, run, punching heavy bag, swim, jump rope or aerobics)

30 minutes of stretching (can even be done while watching TV – calf, hamstring, quad, stomach, arm, shoulder, wrist, neck)

## Wednesday-(weights or bands) - legs & stomach

Round 1–dead lifts
Round 2–squats
Round 3–calf raises
Round 4–lunges
Round 5–side to side shift
Round 6–seated knee lifts
Round 7–seated leg lifts
Round 8–seated bicycle
Round 9–repeat 4–round 2, 3, 7, 6

## Thursday (weights / dumbbells) - back, chest & neck

Round 1–bench press
Round 2–alternating bench press
Round 3–incline bench
Round 4–flys
Round 5–bent over row
Round 6–lawn mower pull
Round 7–staggered push-up
Round 8–tricep push-up
Round 9–repeat 4–round 1, 4, 5, 6

## Friday - walk, hobby & stretching

30-minute walk after dinner and 30 minutes of hobby (walk / hobby – softball, golf, volleyball, tennis)

30 minutes of stretching (while you watch TV – calf, hamstring, quad, stomach, arm, shoulder, wrist, neck)

## Saturday Special - full body cardio and weights combo

2min. Exercise + 1 min. Isometric
(keep a record of the number of reps that you complete and try to improve upon it each Saturday)

Round 1–2 minutes–push ups
Round 1–1 minute isometric–horse stance
Round 2–2 minutes–squats
Round 2–1 minute isometric–jockey stance
Round 3–2 minutes–clean and press
Round 3–1 minute isometric–horse stance
Round 4–2 minutes–jumps
Round 4–1 minute isometric–jockey stance
Round 5- 2 minutes–dead lift

Round 5–1 minute isometric–horse stance
Round 6–2 minutes–jumping jacks
Round 6–1 minute isometric–jockey stance
Round 7–2 minutes–v sit-ups
Round 7–1 minute isometric–horse stance
Round 8–2 minutes–leg flutter
Round 8–1 minute isometric–jockey stance
Round 9–2 minutes–mountain climber
Round 9–1 minute isometric–horse stance

## Sunday - walk, hobby & stretching

30-minute walk after dinner and 30 minutes of hobby (walk / hobby – softball, golf, volleyball, tennis)

30 minutes of stretching (calf, hamstring, quad, stomach, arm, shoulder, wrist, neck)

# Week five through twelve:

Repeat the steps for weeks 1-4 for another two months. After three months of alternating these routines you will be stronger, more toned and have a noticed increase in your stamina and energy. After the first three months you might want to start the twelve week process again or adapt it to your own liking. Consider doing an entire month of stamina (week 4 exercises) or build more muscle by using more weight and repeating week 3 for an entire month. Whatever routine you choose to adopt, make sure that you stay consistent and at least do something!

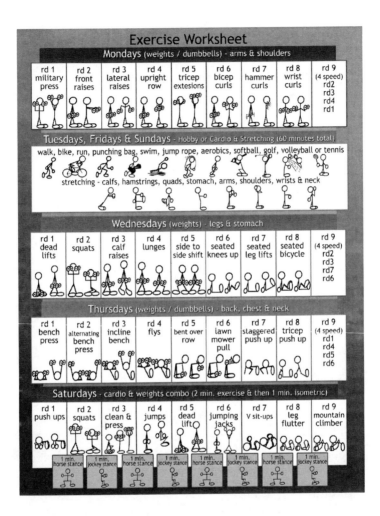

# Exercise Worksheet

## Mondays (weights / dumbbells) - arms & shoulders

| rd 1 military press | rd 2 front raises | rd 3 lateral raises | rd 4 upright row | rd 5 tricep extesions | rd 6 bicep curls | rd 7 hammer curls | rd 8 wrist curls | rd 9 (4 speed) rd2 rd3 rd4 rd1 |
|---|---|---|---|---|---|---|---|---|

## Tuesdays, Fridays & Sundays - Hobby or Cardio & Stretching (60 minutes total)

walk, bike, run, punching bag, swim, jump rope, aerobics, softball, golf, volleyball or tennis

stretching - calfs, hamstrings, quads, stomach, arms, shoulders, wrists & neck

## Wednesdays (weights) - legs & stomach

| rd 1 dead lifts | rd 2 squats | rd 3 calf raises | rd 4 lunges | rd 5 side to side shift | rd 6 seated knees up | rd 7 seated leg lifts | rd 8 seated bicycle | rd 9 (4 speed) rd2 rd3 rd7 rd6 |
|---|---|---|---|---|---|---|---|---|

## Thursdays (weights / dumbbells) - back, chest & neck

| rd 1 bench press | rd 2 alternating bench press | rd 3 incline bench | rd 4 flys | rd 5 bent over row | rd 6 lawn mower pull | rd 7 staggered push up | rd 8 tricep push up | rd 9 (4 speed) rd1 rd4 rd5 rd6 |
|---|---|---|---|---|---|---|---|---|

## Saturdays - cardio & weights combo (2 min. exercise & then 1 min. isometric)

| rd 1 push ups | rd 2 squats | rd 3 clean & press | rd 4 jumps | rd 5 dead lift | rd 6 jumping jacks | rd 7 V sit-ups | rd 8 leg flutter | rd 9 mountain climber |
|---|---|---|---|---|---|---|---|---|
| 1 min. horse stance | 1 min. jockey stance | 1 min. horse stance | 1 min. jockey stance | 1 min. horse stance | 1 min. jockey stance | 1 min. horse stance | 1 min. jockey stance | |

# Dining Out, Celebrations and Eating at a Friend's House

*T*hree of the easiest places to stumble when trying to maintain a new healthy eating lifestyle are when you go out to a restaurant, eat at a friend's house, or attend a celebration of some kind. These are all places that you get out of your comfort zone because someone else is preparing the food for you. The key to all of these situations is controlling your portion sizes, which we will detail and teach you later, but you can also take control of special celebrations by utilizing just a few simple tips.

In all three of these situations (dining out, celebrations, eating at a friend's house), our recommendation is to eat a handful of mixed nuts and drink a large glass of water before you attend the event. The water will help to provide some bulk in your stomach so you aren't as tempted to overeat, and the healthy fats and proteins in the nuts will satisfy your body's craving for nutrients. Have you ever noticed that when you eat at a fast food restaurant you're hungry again an hour or two later? That's because your body is craving nutrients and all that you've given it are empty calories. The oil that they used to fry the potatoes in might have made them taste really good but they provided no benefit for your body. Remember that your body is a field and you are the farmer. Whatever you plant is what you'll harvest. Most fast food is processed and lacks nutrients, so a few hours later your stomach is saying, "excuse me. If you're not too busy up there I really would enjoy it if you could send room service down here with a multitude of morsels." You can try to ignore your stomach but it will start to get impatient and make noises or send little reminders to you by way of cramps. Since your visit to fast food provided no nutrition you give in to the demands of your stomach and load more calories into your field and then wonder why you can't fit into those pants that you bought last month.

Your body will let you know when it needs fuel and nuts are a great way to get a small snack and boost of nutrients that can carry you over for several hours. That's also why they are a great precursor to prepare you for dining out or eating a meal that someone else prepared.

We promised to walk you through three areas that you might stumble or be tempted, so we'll address dining out at a restaurant first. Hopefully you've already prepared yourself ahead of time by downing a glass or two of water at home and snacking on a handful of nuts. So the next thing to do is to avoid the bread, chips, or any of the other temptations that sneak onto your table before the meal. If you simply can't control yourself and the breadsticks and dipping sauce seem to call to you by name, then politely tell the server that you don't care for any and ask if they wouldn't mind removing it from the table. It really is that simple. It's no different than turning the channel on your TV when something offensive comes on or walking out of a movie if they blaspheme God. You do have a choice, so choose to remove the temptation (bread or chips) or remove yourself from the situation. We better move on before we start preaching a sermon on remaining righteous by honoring God in all aspects of your life by protecting your eyes and ears from the immoral onslaught of Hollywood.

Ordering your meal is the next hurdle. Don't be afraid to ask the server to prepare something in a special way or see if they can substitute some of the side dishes. Even if it costs an extra dollar to have steamed broccoli instead of cheese and butter smothered mashed potatoes, it's worth it. You can also ask them to put the dressing for your salad on the side, that way you control how much to put on. The dressing for your salad can often double the amount of calories, so use it sparingly. You also want to be careful with the sauces. Try getting your fish without the creamy sauce or ask for it on the side as well.

When your server does bring the main dish, be cautious because restaurants are notorious for serving portion sizes that are much more than you need. As soon as they bring out the meal, immediately ask for a to-go container.

Now divide your portions in half and put one of those halves into the container and close the lid. Now you won't be tempted to eat more than you should and you have a second meal for tomorrow so you actually got two meals for the price of one. We know, you're thinking, there is no way that you would ask for a to-go container right away. What would the server think of you? What about the other people that might see you and what will they think? Let us put this as delicately as we can; *who cares* what they think! If someone is going to criticize you for taking care of yourself, then they have an issue and it's their problem, not yours. You might need to remind yourself that you are living a life to please God by taking care of His temple of the Holy Spirit. You shouldn't be living a life looking for the approval of others, let alone a stranger at a restaurant. If they're going to criticize you for something as insignificant and petty as dividing your meal, then they're going to criticize you for just about anything anyway. Don't waste even one second worrying about what they might think. If it's a major issue with you then we suggest that you tap into the boldness that you used in the grocery store to avoid the chips on isle three, and announce to your waiter in a voice just loud enough for the table of on-lookers at your left to hear, "Thank you, mister waiter, a buy-one-get-one-free meal, what a blessing you are to us." Then don't be surprised if that same table that was judging you is now asking their waiter how your table got a free meal. You might even start a new to-go container trend just by taking one simple step of controlling your portion sizes.

One of the main things that we can encourage you to do when dining out is to treat your server with respect. You might even consider tipping them double what is recommended, and then don't be surprised if the next time that you go to that restaurant the same server might ask you if you want bread on the table instead of automatically bringing it, or they might ask you if you want a to-go container to come out when they bring your meal. Goodness and mercy will follow you if you treat others the way that Jesus commands us.

Finally, skip dessert or if you absolutely just have to have one, split it among everyone at the table and only take two bites. For each bite, chew it for at least 15-20 seconds and savor the flavor. Those two bites will last a long time and should satisfy your desire for something sweet; plus you've only consumed 40-50 calories instead of the 500-600 if you ate the entire thing.

You can use several of these same techniques if you're going to eat at a friend's house. Thirty-three percent of Americans are classified as obese and the number of people that want to lose weight is far greater than that. If you share your new desire to live a healthier life with your friends then they should be understanding and welcoming, so don't be afraid to be open about your new desire. You won't offend them if you explain how many calories are in dressing and why you put it on the side and just add a small amount for a little taste. Another fun thing to do is to talk to them about portion sizes and how the food industry has changed over the years (reference the chapter on "Portion Sizes" for industry details).

The main point that we want you to grasp when eating at a restaurant or visiting a friend's house is that it's your field that you are taking care of. You need to take responsibility for yourself. There is absolutely nothing wrong with saying, "No thank you, I'm trying to avoid that because I've made a new commitment to be healthier." If someone doesn't respect that then they probably aren't a true friend or a decent restaurant anyway. If they know that you're trying to eat healthier then they should do everything that they can to help you. Would they offer a drink to a recovering alcoholic? We hope not, so they shouldn't offer something unhealthy to someone that is trying to adopt new and healthier eating habits.

The third and final location on our list of easy places for you to stumble is a celebration. We need to be perfectly honest with you and share something personal. If you wanted to read a book written by perfect people or someone that has the discipline to make the right eating choice in every situation, then you've probably already figured out that this isn't the book for you. The only perfect person was Jesus so read your Bible and meditate on every word and teaching that he displayed. But as for us, Robert loves sweets and has to remind himself periodically to use caution concerning what he sows into his body, especially when it comes to ice cream or a nice piece of cake. The other day I tried to rationalize having a piece of cake by saying to myself, "This event only comes around once a year, it won't hurt me to have a piece of cake today." Then it dawned on me; how many times each year can I say that? So I started to count the number of special occasions. At first I thought that there were only a few: Christmas, New Year's and birthday. Then I had to be honest with myself and really think about every occasion or encounter where cake or sweets are present. It was shocking! First of all, take into account how many calories there are in your average piece of cake, it's around 300. And it takes 3,600 calories to equal one pound of fat. So keep those numbers handy and compare your list of special occasions with ours, and be honest with yourself, God is watching you.

We don't celebrate everything on this list but we wanted it to be comprehensive so that you get the point that there are unlimited reasons that people get together for special events and telling yourself that a piece of cake just this once won't hurt, well it will hurt because it isn't just once. If you had a piece of cake at every occasion listed below (70), you would consume 21,000 calories, which over one year is 5.8 pounds. Even if you cut the list in half, it's still 10,500 calories and 2.9 pounds. If you're still trying to justify to yourself that your list is no where near that extensive, then consider that even cutting the list down by 1/3 still equals 7,000 calories and 1.94 pounds per year.

One important reminder concerning our list is that it only mentions holidays and celebrations. How often does someone at your office or church bring donuts? Oh it's Friday, so you thought a donut would be okay. That donut can have anywhere from 200-300 calories so if you had one every Friday then you can add another 52 servings to your total for special occasions and that's an additional 10,400 – 15,600 calories, or 2.8 – 4.3 pounds each year. Ouch! One simple donut every Friday can add 3-4 pounds per year! If that doesn't open your eyes and make you think twice before reaching for that icing-covered, artery-clogging belt buster, then you might need to start over at chapter one and pay special attention on how to create something as your "yuck" food. That might not seem that extreme to put on an extra 3-4 pounds, but let's put it into perspective. Over the next five years just one donut per week can add another 14 – 22 pounds to your weight. Now add the once-a-week office donut to your list of special occasions and you can gain anywhere from 28 – 44 pounds in 5 short years. No wonder so many people think that they're eating healthy and can't understand why their clothes don't fit anymore! Just learn to say "no thank you." Most people have very few problems saying no in average, everyday occasions. Remember the car that wanted the same parking place that you think you saw first? No problems saying or thinking *no* in that instance. Or what about the last time your child tugged on your shirt asking if they can have a cookie? Oh sure, no problem saying no to a cookie for a child that you love but you have trouble saying no to a co-worker when they offer you a donut! What about the solicitor that called you and you cut them off to say no even though they were collecting money for a worthwhile missions program. You had no problem rejecting them but you have trouble telling Suzie at the office "no" when she offers you a donut? We certainly have no problem saying no when it concerns other areas of our lives, so practice it when you're offered a donut or cake.

We're not saying to never reward yourself or take part in a special occasion, but here is a healthy alternative.

First of all reduce the list below and make up your mind that you will reward yourself only once per week, and you do that with a piece of dark chocolate (not white or milk chocolate, it has to be dark chocolate). Most people crave chocolate when they want something sweet anyway, so make it dark and limit yourself to 1-2 ounces, not an entire bar. You also want to make sure that your dark chocolate is at least 65% cocoa content, and avoid most commercial brands that add fat and sugars. It's the same mindset as your portion size. If you can change your routine and habits and encourage those around you to do the same, then it will benefit you, your friends and all of your loved ones. Instead of ordering a cake for that special occasion, present a tray of individual pieces of dark chocolate, you can even stick a candle in some of them to blow out.

Our advice to eat a small piece of dark chocolate isn't a license to eat candy bars, because a 100 gram candy bar has 480 calories, and you would have to reduce your calorie count that day to counter that, so just a few ounces once per week is perfect. There's nothing wrong with not eating cake at two parties that week because you know that you're going to have your dark chocolate this weekend as a reward. Don't give in to the immediate satisfaction and temptation of that icing covered cake. Look forward to the reward at the end of the week, which is your small piece of dark chocolate and your longer term reward: a healthier field. Wow, that's a pretty powerful allegory for our everyday walk. Avoid the temptations of the enemy and the world, and look toward the prize at the end; heaven and our eternal salvation.

How does your list stack up against this one, and be honest?

*Special Occasion list:*

- ___my birthday
- ___spouse's birthday
- ___wedding anniversary
- ___child #1's birthday
- ___child #2's birthday
- ___mother's birthday
- ___father's birthday
- ___brother's birthday
- ___sister's birthday
- ___niece #1's birthday
- ___nephew #1's birthday
- ___niece #2's birthday
- ___nephew #2's birthday
- ___boss' birthday

- ___fellow employees & friends birthdays = 18 (everyone has a birthday; how many people do you know?)

- ___New Year's Eve

- ___New Year's Day

- ___Epiphany

- ___Martin Luther King Jr. Day

- ___Chinese New Year

- ___Groundhog Day

- ___Valentine's Day

- ___President's Day

- ___Fat Tuesday

- ___St. Patrick's Day

- ___first day of spring

- ___April Fool's Day

- ___Palm Sunday

- ___Passover

- ___Good Friday

- ___Easter

- ___Earth Day

- ___Arbor Day
- ___May Day
- ___Mother's Day
- ___Memorial Day
- ___Flag Day
- ___Father's Day
- ___Emancipation Day
- ___Independence Day – 4th of July
- ___Labor Day
- ___Rosh Hashanah
- ___Yom Kipper
- ___Columbus Day
- ___All Saints' Day
- ___Veteran's Day
- ___Thanksgiving Day
- ___Thanksgiving leftovers
- ___Thanksgiving leftovers, leftover
- ___Hanukkah
- ___Christmas Eve

- ___Christmas Day

- ___Christmas leftovers

We realize that you may not celebrate even one third of these, especially considering that we have Christmas and Hanukkah on the same list, but it's designed to make you think of how many opportunities there are each year that you may be presented with a piece of celebratory cake.

If you're at a celebration and you absolutely have to have some Birthday or Anniversary cake, then use our tip from earlier and take time to chew. Instead of eating the entire piece of cake, *only* take two bites. Chew each bite for 15 seconds and casually observe others while you're chewing. You will probably notice that in the 30 seconds it takes you to finish just two bites, there will be several people that will consume an entire piece of cake in that same amount of time. They wolf down 10 or 15 bites so fast that they didn't get to enjoy the taste as much as you did. If you want to have some fun with this, keep a log of how many times each week you are at an occasion where cake is served or you are offered a donut. You might be surprised at the total. If you have any role in an event, try our tip on having just 1-2 ounces (everything in moderation) of dark chocolate. If anyone has an issue with your attempt to offer a healthier alternative, place a 4-pound can of lard next to your small piece of chocolate on the table with a sign explaining that this is how many pounds of fat cake can add to your body in just one year. If you don't want to be that extreme, you could always place a card next to your dessert listing the benefits of 1-2 ounces of dark chocolate (not an entire candy bar). The main ingredient of chocolate is cocoa, which has been shown in research to reduce blood pressure, reduce cell damage and even reduce the risk of heart disease.

We hope that you will be able to take and use these tools when dining out, celebrating a special occasion, or eating at a friend's house. Each time that you see a donut or piece of cake, you can always picture your "yuck" food (from Chapter #3) and you should have no problem avoiding it, or think about what kind of a harvest it will yield. If you plant sugar from donuts and cake into your body, you're going to yield what you've sown and ruin a lot of the hard work that you put in all week tending to your field. One to two ounces of dark chocolate won't ruin your field, it can easily melt off of your tractor, but two donuts will clog up your gas tank.

# Your Hands Hold the Key-Portion Sizes

We spent the first few sections of this book outlining most of the major obstacles that prevent you from achieving a healthy weight and we hope that you are encouraged to change your routine, resist temptation, and find healthier options when shopping or snacking. Now we are going to address what we consider to be the biggest obstacle standing in your way and that's portion sizes. Obesity has become an epidemic in America and our export of fast food restaurants to the rest of the world is impacting all of those nations as well. If you look at portion sizes throughout the history of America, there has been an explosion in the last 50–60 years. The average cup of coffee in the '50's was only about 5 ounces. Today, there is a popular coffee chain whose smallest size is 12 ounces, which is called a tall but we don't have the time or space in this book to rant about how ridiculous and what an oxymoron it is to call your small size a tall. The next two sizes at that same establishment are 16 and 20 ounces. That's three to four times as large as what our grandparents drank.

If you're starting to drift off because you tire of people talking about the "good old days," we need you to focus for just one more minute because these upcoming numbers are quite shocking and might help to explain why the average adult is 26 pounds heavier than they were in 1950's. According to new figures released by the Center for Disease Control the average restaurant meal is now four times larger than it was in the 1950's. In the 50's, the average hamburger was 3.9 ounces. It's now at 12 ounces. French fries went from 2.4 ounces to almost 7 ounces. [6] What about sodas? Do you remember the little tiny bottles from the 50's, they averaged about 7 ounces compared to the 64-ounce monsters that people flood themselves with these days. If that isn't shocking enough, look at a cookbook from the 50's and you'll be astonished that the standard pasta measurement was 1 ½ cups while most restaurants today use up to 3 cups. Even a tray of brownies in the 50's would be cut into 24 squares whereas today they'll be sliced into only 9 or 12.

If you really compare and study those numbers, it's no wonder that obesity has become the leading health risk in the United States today. You might not think of obesity as a larger threat than some of the more recognizable diseases, but look at some of the health risks associated with obesity: cancer, depression, gallbladder disease, gynecological problems such as infertility and irregular periods, heart disease, high blood pressure, metabolic syndrome, nonalcoholic fatty liver disease, osteoarthritis, intertrigo skin problems, impaired wound healing, sleep apnea, stroke and type 2 diabetes.

So the era of super sizing meals, glorification of hot dog eating contests as a sport, and restaurants that offer a free 72 ounce steak if you can eat it in one hour, have all come with a costly price tag: the health of America. One in three adults is now considered obese. So the next time you're at church, look to your left, then to your right, and the odds are that one of you is obese. If the people on either side of you appear to be really thin, then guess who the one out of three is, it must be you! Just kidding. Don't look around at others. This book is about you making a declaration to start taking better care of yourself, addressing the plank in your own eye, not judging others.

Hopefully we've made our point that portion sizes play one of the key roles in controlling your weight. Well God has given you the tool to help you eat the proper portion sizes and it's something that you take with you everywhere you go. You don't need to carry a special book around or keep Tupperware containers in your purse for measuring. No need to pull a small scale out at the restaurant or count how many green beans you're allowed to have at lunch. God has put the power in your own hands to quickly and easily manage your portion sizes. Literally, He has put the knowledge and wisdom in your hands. He has given you a hand in making your choices. We have to hand it to Him. This simple portion size measuring cup is really handy. Enough already! We can't take any more corny metaphors. Your *hands* are the key.

God deals in perfect creation and your hands form the perfect portion size plate, and that plate is even partitioned for you by God to show you how much of each food group the individual segments should contain. We're going to show you how to divide your hands into six different food segments and eat the perfect amount of each group utilizing your new found portion plate. Think of your hands as if they were the separated segments of a TV dinner. Don't get overwhelmed, it's going to be as easy as painting by numbers. There's also no need to panic and think that a meal the size of your hands will starve you! If you eat three meals per day using your portion-size hands, it will equal the perfect amount to help you achieve and maintain a healthy weight. For our example we're going to use around 1,500 calories which is almost the perfect amount for a female that weighs around 115 pounds. If you compare a 115 pound woman's hands to those of a man that weighs 220 pounds, you'll quickly notice that the man's hands are quite a bit larger. The thickness of your hands also determines the portion size. For your poultry, the piece should be the thickness of your palm so the 115 pound woman might have a 3 ounce piece but the 220 pound man's palm would be closer to 4-5 ounces. If you have extremely large hands, then the remainder of your body should be proportional in size so you'll need more calories anyway. Each person's hands in your family should be just right for themselves. You don't have to worry about carrying separate special measuring devices for each family member; God provided it for each one of us.

This new portion size plate also helps us prove our point on how unhealthy fast food can be. Try an experiment for us and buy one large order of French Fries at your local fast food restaurant. Now pour that entire order into your hands and you'll notice that it covers every section of your new portion plate. What we've reserved for all six food groups and your whole meal is overwhelmed by just one portion of unhealthy fried food. It's no wonder obesity is plaguing our country and having such a detrimental effect on our children.

So how should you fill your newly discovered God-given portion plate? Let's divide your hands into the different food categories and we'll explain how it works. Start by cupping your hands together like you're trying to contain some water that you just scooped out of a cool Colorado stream. Take a really good look at how they are divided up and the size of each section. If you're still holding this book then you haven't taken a look. Go ahead, place the book down for just a second and cup your hands together; that's your portion plate.

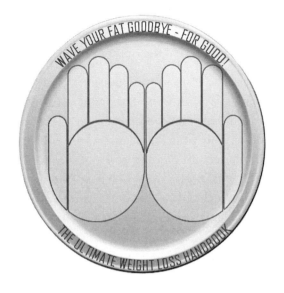

Now we'll divide your hands into 6 segments: your palms, fingers and thumbs. We're also going to use catchy names for each portion segment to make it easier for you to remember. We find that memorization and recall are much easier if you can attach a fun name and a visual image to that item. Therefore, we've come up with an almost childlike name and image for each segment of your hands so that even if you're rushing around trying to prepare your very first dinner for your in-laws, you will still easily be able to remember how much pasta you should serve.

# Poultry Palm

*L*et's start on the left most side by looking at your palm. This is the portion size for your protein, so we could call it your protein palm, but since chicken and turkey are such a great source for protein, we like to call this your Poultry Palm. Say it slowly and annunciate, Poultry Palm. It's not a Poetry Palm; that would be some strange form of writing on your hand. It's a Poultry Palm.

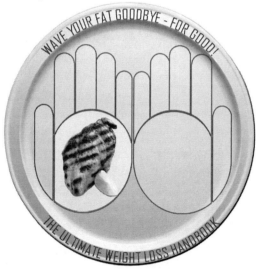

If you ignore your thumb and fingers and focus just on the palm area, it's the perfect size for your protein. If you fill it with a piece of fish or turkey, it will be about 4 ounces, which is exactly what you need. Keep in mind that you get that much protein for three meals so your daily total will be 12 ounces which is more than enough. You might even consider only using your poultry palm for two meals and doubling up on fruits and vegetables for breakfast instead, but we'll cover that in our fourteen day menu that we lay out for you later. We also want to encourage you to be creative with your protein. Don't be afraid to use foods like eggs or legumes.

Here is a list of some foods that you can use for your protein: black-eyed peas, bean burgers, black beans, chicken, chickpeas (garbanzo beans), dry beans, eggs, falafel, garden burgers, ham, kidney beans, lamb, lean beef, lentils, lima beans (mature), navy beans, peanut butter, peas, pinto beans, soy beans, split peas, tempeh, texturized vegetable protein (TVP), tofu (bean curd made from soybeans), turkey, veggie burgers & white beans.

We also have a great list of seafood that is a fantastic source of protein: anchovies, cod, flounder, haddock, halibut, herring, mackerel, pollock, porgy, salmon, sardines, scallops, sea bass, snapper, swordfish, trout & tuna.

Your Poultry Palm is vitally important to your daily meals as you continue to adopt new hobbies, develop a habit of walking after meals, and stay consistent with your exercise routines. Protein will be the key in helping to fuel your body and rebuild your muscles, especially as you start to get toward those middle age years. Once we reach 40 years of age our muscle mass begins to deteriorate at 10% per decade, so you must stay active and get the proper amounts of protein to build up your health and counteract the effects of aging. Look at your left palm one more time; it's your protein portion-size plate that will now be known as your Poultry (or protein) Palm.

# Fruit Fingers

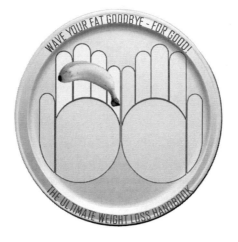

WAVE YOUR FAT GOODBYE - FOR GOOD!

THE ULTIMATE WEIGHT LOSS HANDBOOK

We covered the palm of your left hand; now move up that same hand to your fingers. God created your fingers as the perfect measuring tool for your fruits. So we call them your Fruit Fingers. When your hand is cupped your fingers actually look kind of like a small bunch of bananas anyway, so that's an easy way to remember it. If you have an apple, some grapes, or cut a banana in half, they should fit perfectly into the portion-size space of your left hand fingers. One of the best things about your fruits is that you can substitute them for some of your other food groups if you want to, particularly for breakfast. You could have a smoothie that represents several different portion sizes and skip your protein or vegetables that morning.

Many of us get into a habit of eating the same few food types so we want to give you a list of fruits so that you can experiment and try all of them at some point so that you can discover new tastes while you're discovering new things about your own ability to conquer those old fears about getting healthier.

Here are several different fruits including many that you may have never tried so we encourage you to be adventurous and creative: Apples, Apricots, Avocado, Bananas, Blueberries, Cantaloupe, Cherries, Grapefruit, Grapes, Honeydew, Kiwi, Lemons, Limes, Mangoes, Nectarines, Oranges, Papaya, Peaches, Pears, Pineapple, Plums, Prunes, Raisins, Raspberries, Strawberries, Tangerines and Watermelon.

When was the last time that you had Kiwi or Papaya? If it's been a while, then step back up to the plate and add some variety to your meals.

# Fat Finger

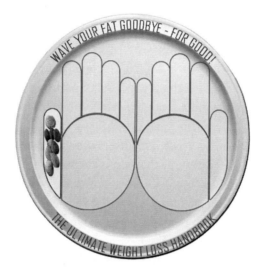

WAVE YOUR FAT GOODBYE - FOR GOOD!

THE ULTIMATE WEIGHT LOSS HANDBOOK

We've covered your left Poultry Palm and Fruit Fingers, now it's over to your left thumb. We call it your Fat Finger. It represents how much oil and fat you should have. It truly is a fat finger so it should be one of the easier of the six portion segments to remember. A Fat Finger for your fats, how much more straightforward could it be. Oil and fats represent several different foods, everything from the oil you use in your skillet to mixed nuts as a snack. Here is a list of foods that constitute your oil and fats food group. Any time that you prepare your meal, look at your left thumb, your Fat Finger, and that's your portion size.

Fats & oils: almonds, avocados, butter, cashews, canola oil, corn oil, cottonseed oil, hazelnuts, mixed nuts, olive oil, peanuts, pecans, pistachios, pumpkin seeds, safflower oil, sesame seeds, soybean oil, sunflower oil, sunflower seeds, olives and walnuts.

Not all of those fats are healthy fats, but if you absolutely have to cook with something like butter, then limit it to the size of your fat finger. Your left thumb isn't very big is it? That's exactly the point. It's a simple way to know how many pistachios to have. Instead of eating the entire bag, a small grouping the size of your thumb is perfect. The interesting thing about fats is that there are some that are considered healthy fats. Olive oil has a lot of calories but is considered to be much better than butter. Avocados are extremely high in calories as well but they contain over 20 vitamins and are fantastic for you. The benefits of most natural fruits and vegetables far outweigh the negative count of the calories. It's the processed foods that you need to try and stay away from. Especially things like margarine that has trans fats. Make sure and read the label so you know what you're putting into your body.

There are several different kinds of fats which can make it confusing so we're going to give you a quick breakdown to better explain it. The American Heart Association is a great resource for you to look up more information, so we're going to site some of their research for you. The four main fats that we want to detail are saturated, trans, monounsaturated and polyunsaturated.

Saturated fats occur naturally in many foods like fatty beef, poultry skin, butter and cheese just to outline a few. Many fried foods also contain high levels of saturated fats. These fats can raise your cholesterol and increase your risk of heart disease and stroke so avoid them or minimize your exposure as much as possible. That's why it's a good practice to not eat the skin of the chicken.

Trans fats are the next danger zone. They are created in an industrial process that is inexpensive to produce and prolongs the shelf life of an item. They also increase the texture and taste of the food and can be used multiple times in a fryer so they are a favorite for many restaurants. Trans fats, also called partially hydrogenated oils, raise your bad cholesterol (LDL) and lower your good cholesterol (HDL) levels as well as increase your risk of heart disease, stroke, and developing type 2 diabetes. Trans fats can be found in French fries, donuts, pizza dough, cookies and stick margarine.

The Food and Drug Administration (FDA) requires that all foods list trans fats on their nutrition fact panel as long as it is more than .5 grams per serving. So read the label carefully because if they consider half a cookie to be one serving, then they might be able to list the trans fats at 0 grams even though an entire cookie could have .9 grams. If it lists partially hydrogenated oil, then it contains trans fats and you might consider putting it back on the shelf. Keep in mind that the FDA regulation only applies to packaged foods, not food that is served in a restaurant, bakery or grocery store.

The final two fats, which are the healthy replacements for trans and saturated, are monounsaturated and polyunsaturated. The key to using these as replacements is moderation. Use your "fat finger" as your guide. These healthy fats help reduce bad cholesterol, contain several nutrients and are high in vitamin E and antioxidants. Monounsaturated fats include canola oil, olive oil, peanut oil, sesame oil and sunflower oil as well as avocados, nuts and peanut butter.

Polyunsaturated fats are also very beneficial including omega 3 and omega 6 fats which play a crucial role in your brain function. That should get your attention! Foods high in polyunsaturated fats include corn oil, safflower oil, soybean oil, sunflower seeds, vegetable oil, walnuts, as well as fatty fish like salmon and trout.[7]

We've listed four fats for you so to keep it straight, remember the bad fats are saturated, trans and partially hydrogenated oil (which is another name for trans fats). The two that are good for you are the only ones with *un* in them; monounsaturated and polyunsaturated. Just remember the *un* and you'll be safe. Don't let partially hydrogenated oil throw you by saying that it's an oil and try to confuse you into thinking that olive oil is good so this oil must be good. If it doesn't have the *un*, it's not safe. The *un* keeps it safe.

Here are a few simple things to try when thinking about your fat finger. Instead of loading your bread (which should be whole wheat or rye and never regular white) with butter or mayonnaise, try hummus or a little olive oil instead. And for that old family recipe that requires an entire stick of butter, replace it with half of the suggested ingredient and try using olive oil or find a light butter that is part olive oil. The more natural the product the more healthy fat that it usually contains. So try and use more natural products and less processed foods, for example: the fat in a finger size portion of pecans is much better for you than a tablespoon of peanut butter. Most peanut butters add trans fats and other additives that are more detrimental than the positive fats from the peanuts themselves. So choose the natural alternative whenever possible. Your pledge is to start sowing healthier seed into your field, so make sure that you sow as much natural seed as you can, especially when it comes to fats. Instead of saying that you are naturally fat, start saying that you will sow natural fats. There is a big difference in those two statements. One is an excuse and the other is a new pledge of health.

# Pasta Palm

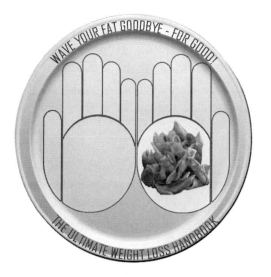

WAVE YOUR FAT GOODBYE - FOR GOOD!

THE ULTIMATE WEIGHT LOSS HANDBOOK

*Y*our left hand is now full of fruits (fingers), poultry (palm) and nuts (fat finger), so let's move on to your right hand starting with your palm. This is your portion size area for your grains, so we call it the Pasta Palm. We know, it's a corny rhyme but it should make it easier to remember. There have been so many books and diets written about avoiding pasta, staying away from carbohydrates of any kind, but we encourage you to eat whole grain or whole wheat for your pastas. Here is a very *important note*! You need to be cautious of what the main banner on the box or packaging claims, because that is their marketing ploy. It might say 100% whole wheat, but that might not tell the entire story. The whole wheat that they use might be 100%, but what if only 20% of the product is whole wheat and 80% is refined or enriched flour? How can you be sure what you're buying? Read the ingredients. The FDA has mandated that every product must list the ingredients in descending order of quantity in the product. If the first ingredient is whole grain, then you know that it is the dominant ingredient. If the first ingredient listed is refined flour, then make a mental note to put a sign on that product that states, "Danger – do not enter my field." Make sure that you read the label for everything that you put into your grocery cart!

As you start to read the ingredients on more and more products, you will notice that enriched and refined grains are listed for many types of pasta. Refined grains are the ones that you want to try to completely avoid. The refining process strips so many of the vitamins that it might be healthier for you to eat the box! Of course we're kidding, but since you have an option then why not choose something healthier like whole wheat or whole grain.

In addition to seeing the phrase refined grains, you will also see what is called enriched. That's because many refined grains are enriched. This means that certain B vitamins (thiamin, riboflavin, niacin, folic acid) and iron are added back after processing. So enriched is better than refined, but fiber is not added back to the enriched grains.

Many food products are made from mixtures of whole grains and refined grains so check the ingredient list on every product that you purchase and pay special attention to the order that the ingredients are listed so that you know what the most dominant ingredients are. Look for whole grain or whole wheat for all of your pastas and grains.

Here is a list to give you an idea of some grains that you might not be accustomed to eating. Some of these might help your recipe book to grow even larger and add some additional variety to your meals.

Whole grains: amaranth, brown rice, buckwheat, cracked wheat, crackers, millet, muesli, oatmeal, popcorn, quinoa, sorghum, triticale, whole grain barley, whole grain cornmeal, whole wheat bread, whole wheat cereal flakes, whole wheat crackers, whole wheat pasta, whole wheat sandwich buns & rolls, whole wheat tortillas, whole rye and wild rice.

Refined grains that you want to try and avoid can include: cornbread, corn flakes, corn tortillas, couscous, crackers (most brands), flour tortillas, grits, noodles, pasta, macaroni, pitas, pretzels, white bread, white sandwich buns, white rolls and white rice.

Most whole grains and whole wheat pastas have a lot more flavor than your standard refined grains anyway, so your taste buds will thank you for making some of these changes. Think about it; a piece of white bread that you could just as easily moisten and use as a papier-mâché project versus a piece of multigrain bread that is full of flavor. Or what about regular spaghetti noodles that stick together on your plate with some form of natural super glue, just as much as they seem to stick to the wall of your stomach. Whole wheat spaghetti noodles have so much more flavor that you won't need to add butter to the noodles just to make them palatable. Try substituting some of our recommendations and create your own new mouth-watering specialties.

# Veggie Fingers

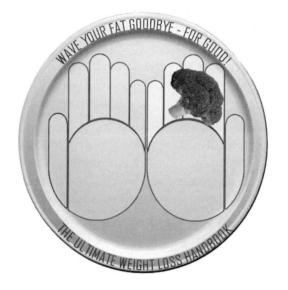

WAVE YOUR FAT GOODBYE - FOR GOOD!

THE ULTIMATE WEIGHT LOSS HANDBOOK

The fifth portion size that God has created and given to you are the fingers on your right hand. These are for your vegetables or what we'll call your Veggie Fingers. If you have trouble getting your children to eat vegetables, try cutting them into slices and calling them veggie fingers. It will make it more fun for them and they are already conditioned by the millions of marketing dollars spent by fast food restaurants to want chicken fingers, so piggyback off of that and encourage them to eat your homemade veggie fingers.

One of the unique things about this portion size is that you can make these your universal coverall and default. That means that you can substitute vegetables for any of your other portion sizes. You might decide to have a complete vegetable lunch and not have any grains or protein. Or include some protein on your salad with a piece of fish, some lean turkey or even just a few cashews, almonds and pecans. The key to this protein salad is to go extremely light on the salad dressing. Spend an extra 20 minutes one day at the grocery store or go on-line and read several of the salad dressing labels until you find a low fat version that you enjoy. You might find a low fat raspberry vinaigrette that is perfect. Then remember your Fat Finger and only add that much dressing which should only be about a tablespoon, not a giant soup ladle portion.

An easy way to ensure that you're getting a good variety of nutrients is to make your meal as colorful as possible and vegetables are a fantastic way to add color to any meal. The more color and the darker the color, the better. Some dark green broccoli, dark red beets and orange butternut squash will make your plate look like Joseph's coat and the amount of nutrients will be a blessing to your field.

Here is a list so that you can add even more new ideas to your recipe book.

- Dark green vegetables: bok choy, broccoli, collard greens, dark green leafy lettuce, kale, mesclun, mustard greens, romaine lettuce, spinach, turnip greens and watercress.

- Orange vegetables: acorn squash, butternut squash, carrots, hubbard squash, pumpkin and sweet potatoes.

- Additional vegetables: artichokes, asparagus, bean sprouts, beets, Brussels sprouts, cabbage, cauliflower, celery, cucumbers, eggplant, green beans, green or red peppers, mushrooms, okra, onions, parsnips, tomato juice, tomatoes, turnips, vegetable juice, wax beans & zucchini.

# Dairy Digit

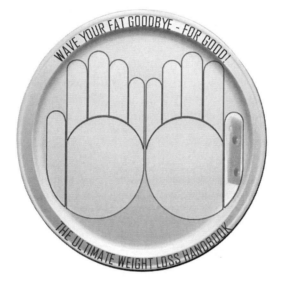

WAVE YOUR FAT GOODBYE - FOR GOOD!

THE ULTIMATE WEIGHT LOSS HANDBOOK

he final of your six food segments is your right thumb. We call this one your Dairy Digit. An easy way to remember this one is that it looks a little bit like a cow utter anyway. Maybe that's why kids suck their thumbs? Did we really just write that your thumb looks like a cow utter and then say something about kids? Yes, we did. We just wanted to make sure that you are paying attention and give you a simple point of reference to remember your dairy digit. Now the next time you see someone milking a cow or a child sucking their thumb, we hope that you'll say, "Oh yeah, the good ol' Dairy Digit."

Your Dairy Digit represents the portion size for your dairy and cheese. Don't try and switch this with your palm or fingers and eat an entire block of cheese, as tempting as that may be. Remember your pledge and stick to the portion plan. What foods and liquids constitute your Dairy food groups? Here is a list of a few: American cheese, cheddar cheese, chocolate milk, cottage cheese, fat free skim milk, fat free yogurt, frozen yogurt, goat cheese, ice milk, kefir, lactose free milk, lactose reduced milk, low fat 1% milk, low fat yogurt, mozzarella cheese, parmesan cheese, reduced fat 2% milk, reduced fat yogurt, ricotta cheese, whole milk, whole milk yogurt.

That concludes the six segments of your God-given portion plate. The catchy names (or some might say that they're silly names), should help you to remember which area goes with what food group. Honestly, how can you forget the Pasta Palm, Fruit Fingers, or especially the Dairy Digit? It's incredible to think that all of this time your hands carried the key. That God has given us the tools and knowledge to eat healthier; we just need to follow His guidance. Maybe His original design for us was to not use plates in the first place. What if He wanted us to use our hands all this time, to hold our food so that we wouldn't overeat by using plates the size of a garbage can lid? Don't let your children read that part about not using a plate or they might try to blame us for justifying eating with their fingers. We encourage you to spend a few minutes reviewing the six segments again so that you can commit them to memory and at the drop of a hat you can recall exactly what each portion size should be. The final chapter of the book includes a fourteen-day menu as a template for you to see how easy and how filling your portion plate hands can be. Now you have the power and knowledge to never overeat again, to easily control your health and weight through your God given portion plate

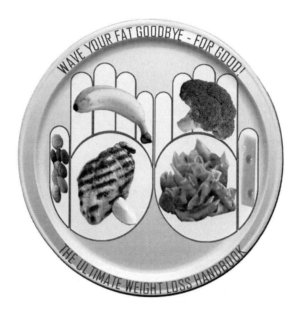

# Prayer Plate

*N*ow that you view your hands in a brand new way, realizing that God actually created a tool for you that will make your life so much easier, there is one more use for them that will help you along your path to a healthier you. Follow along in this simple little exercise. Cup your hands together in the same fashion that you would to determine your proper portion size and then slowly lower your face toward your hands until it is buried in your palms. If you actually put the book down to do this then you can no longer read this page so we don't know how you can follow this next step, but let's assume that you haven't actually buried your face in your palms yet. If you have, go ahead and peek between your fingers to read this next part.

The next step is to pray. Your custom portion size plate that the Lord has given you is also a perfect prayer plate for you to bury your face in as you sing out praise to Him and seek His guidance. One of the most important things you can do on your journey is to talk to Him every day, throughout the day, especially right before a meal. You should bless your food before every meal, and while blessing it, ask the Lord to give you the wisdom to make the right choices in your food selection. If you pray before every meal the Holy Spirit might convict you to put down those super sized fast food fries and grab an apple instead. He has heard you recite your pledge that you "will start sowing the right seed for a healthy harvest!" So as you pray before your meal, don't be surprised if the Holy Spirit speaks to you about your choices. We encourage you to visit your prayer plate as often as you can during the day even when not eating. You don't have to bury your face in your palms when praying, but it can help you to focus and block out distractions. It doesn't matter if you pray while lying on your back with your eyes open, as long as you're praising and seeking Him, He will hear from heaven and answer. If you haven't heard from the Lord recently, or some of you might say that He has never spoken to you, then you need to perform one simple task, read these next two lines.

> Then God said, "Behold I have given you every plant yielding seed that is on the surface of all the earth, and every tree which has fruit yielding seed; it shall be food for you."
>
> Genesis 1:29 (NASB)

> Looking at them, Jesus said, "With people it is impossible, but not with God; for all things are possible with God."
>
> Mark 10:27 (NASB)

There, now you have heard from the Lord. The Bible is the inspired word of God. When you read His word you are hearing from Him. The more you read, memorize and meditate on His word, the more you'll hear from Him. Sowing into your spirit is the same as sowing into your stomach for a healthy harvest. What you feed your spirit through your eyes and ears yields the same results as the seed that you feed your body through your mouth. If you sow horror movies, songs filled with immorality, and images of sin into your eyes and ears; then what do you expect your spirit to harvest? Protect your spirit in the same manner of good harvest that we've been encouraging you to sow into your body. Study the Word, pray and guard your spirit as if your life depended on it, because your afterlife does depend on it.

# Fourteen Days in the Kitchen with Lori

$\mathcal{N}$ ow that we've shown you a simple and effective way to control your portion sizes we want to detail how easy and practical it is to come up with great tasting meals. This fourteen day menu is designed to show you how simple it is to get plenty of nutrients and calories by using your God given portion plate. It is not a recommendation for any readers as a meal plan because we are not physicians or nutritionists, it's simply a 1,500 calorie per day menu that is typical of what Lori might eat over a two week period. Consuming only 1,500 calories per day is a small amount and may not be a healthy option for you depending on your current weight and physical condition. You need to consult with a nutritionist and your physician and get their recommendations on a diet or meal plan that is right for you. Our goal is to show you that by using your hands as a portion plate guide you can have three incredible meals each day, including additional snacks, and still only consume 1,500 calories. That's an entire day of healthy eating and your calorie intake is less than one fast food meal! The best news is that the plan includes a piece of dark chocolate as a reward each weekend so skip the donuts at the office this week and start living a healthier life today!

Before we get started we have two quick tips. Breakfast is important so make your first meal of the day colorful and enjoyable. Also make sure and properly hydrate by including eight glasses of water (8 ounces each) every day. Two with every meal, one before you exercise and another one after you are done exercising.

## Day 1 - total 1,533 calories

Include at least 8 glasses of water–2 with every meal, 1 in the morning and 1 at night

### Breakfast-420 calories-oatmeal with raisins & fruit cup

oatmeal–1 bowl (150)

raisins–1 finger portion size added to oatmeal (120)

cup of fruit-

banana–1 sliced (105)

strawberries–4 large, sliced (45)

### Lunch-351 calories-whole wheat turkey sandwich & an apple

smoked turkey breast (30)

whole wheat bread (100)

Swiss cheese–1 Slice (110)

tomato–2 slices (8)

cucumber–4 slices (8)

apple–1 medium (95)

## Snack-160 calories

organic nut mix – 1 Fat Finger full, 20 pieces (160)

## Dinner-602 calories-spinach salad topped with chicken, vegetable & fruit

baby spinach salad–(10)

roasted chicken–light, protein palm size (242)

strawberries–4 large, chopped (49)

almonds- Fat Finger full, slivers (163)

light vinaigrette fat-free dressing–2 tablespoons (30)

broccoli–steamed (27) with lemon juice (12)

cantaloupe – 1/4 slice (69)

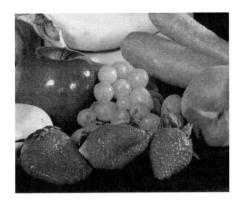

# Day 2-total 1,477 calories

include at least 8 glasses of water–2 with every meal, 1 in the morning and 1 at night

## Breakfast-436 calories-fruit smoothie & English muffin w/ strawberry jelly

Smoothie–frozen unsweetened strawberries (77), low-fat cherry Kefir (174)

whole wheat toasted English muffin (135), 2 tablespoons strawberry jelly (50)

## Lunch-430 calories-tuna stuffed tomato, grapes & herbal tea

tuna–1 can light tuna in water, without salt (191)

tomato–1 whole cut in half (20)

celery–2 sticks raw, cut into small slices (20)

green peas–boiled, drained, w/out salt (62)

carrots–2 large cut into slices (53)

cherry tomatoes–4 cut into slices (22)

Fruit Finger portion full of grapes (62)

1 glass chamomile herbal tea (0)

## Dinner-556 calories-baked chicken with garlic and onions, vegetables & dinner rolls

roasted chicken (266)

cinnamon–ground (6)

onions–boiled, drained without salt (26)

garlic–2 cloves (10)

broccoli–1 cup cooked (27)

cabbage–1 cup cooked (35)

whole wheat dinner rolls–two (76)

olive oil buttery spread–1 tablespoon (60)

## Dessert-105 calories-blended frozen fruit (natural ice treat)

half frozen banana and half an apple blended

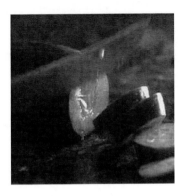

# Day 3-total 1,486 calories

Include at least 8 glasses of water–2 with every meal, 1 in the morning and 1 at night

## Breakfast-411 calories-Mexican omelet & orange juice

eggs–2 scrambled (199)

sliced turkey breast (40)

onions–cooked (26)

peppers–cooked (19)

salsa (15)

orange juice–1 glass (112)

## Lunch -416 calories-black bean burrito, soup & pears

whole wheat tortilla (100)

Swiss cheese -1 slice of 2% low fat (50)

tomato—2 slices (10)

black beans — 1 can of low sodium (110)

chicken vegetable soup (50)

pears—2 sliced (96)

## Snack-95 calories

Apple—1 medium (95)

## Dinner-564 calories-knife and fork turkey burger, new potatoes, broccoli & mixed fruit cup

turkey—fat free, ground (120)

garlic (4)

onions (26)

tomato (22)

sweet peppers (19)

new potatoes (100)

cooked broccoli (27) lemon on broccoli (12)

mixed fruit cup–watermelon (46), blueberries (83), banana (105)

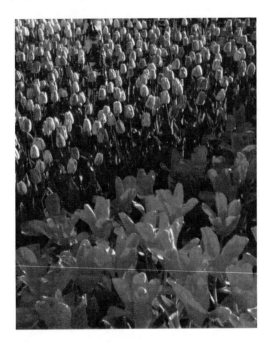

## Day 4-total 1,504 calories

Include at least 8 glasses of water–2 with every meal, 1 in the morning and 1 at night

## Breakfast-377 calories-egg wrap & grapefruit

whole wheat tortilla wrap (76)

eggs–2 scrambled (204)

onions–cooked (26)

peppers–cooked (19)

half a grapefruit (52)

## Lunch-599 calories-spinach salad with fruit and almonds, celery with peanut butter

baby spinach salad (20)

cucumber–1 sliced (8)

apple–1 sliced (95)

grapes–1/3 of your Fruit Fingers full, sliced (62)

strawberries–1/3 of your Fruit Fingers full, sliced (49)

almond–slivers (163)

celery–2 sticks (13)

peanut butter–without salt, 2 tablespoons (189)

## Snack-l05 calories

Banana (105)

## Dinner-423 calories-spaghetti, salad & fruit

whole wheat spaghetti–Pasta Palm full (174)

marinara sauce–Pasta Palm full (70)

parmesan cheese–Dairy Digit portion (42)

romaine lettuce–Veggie Fingers full (15)

cucumber – 1/2 sliced (8)

carrots–1 sliced (53)

red onion–1 sliced (26)

cantaloupe – 1/4 sliced (35)

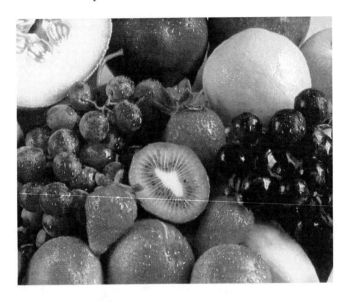

# Day 5-total 1,506 calories

Include at least 8 glasses of water = 2 with every meal, 1 in the morning and 1 at night

## Breakfast-581 calories-turkey & egg muffin, banana, orange juice

whole wheat English muffin – one (135)

egg–1 fried (90)

turkey sausage–1 patty (89)

Swiss cheese–1 slice of 2% low fat (50)

banana (105)

orange juice–1 cup (112)

## Lunch-333 calories-chili, mixed fruits & vegetables

chili–1 bowl (202)

celery stalks–x 4 (11)

carrots–½ cup slices (25)

apple–1 med. (95)

## Dinner-592 calories-roasted chicken over wild rice, mixed vegetables & fruit

roasted chicken – protein palm portion (266)

wild rice–1 cup (166)

mixed vegetables (80)

pears–half a cup (47)

peach–half a cup (33)

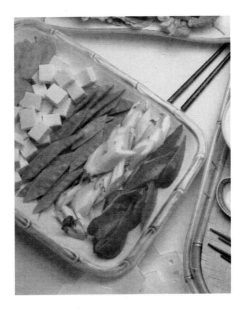

# Day 6-total 1,521 calories

Include at least 8 glasses of water = 2 with every
meal, 1 in the morning and 1 at night

## Breakfast-525 calories-French toast with mixed fruit

2 slices French toast–w/ 2% milk and whole
wheat bread (298)

topped with strawberries (49)

topped with blueberries (83)

apple (95)

## Lunch-405 calories-chicken breast sandwich, pineapple & cottage cheese

whole wheat bread (100)

chicken breast slice (86)

Dijon mustard (5)

low-fat cottage cheese (102)

pineapple added to cottage cheese (78)

carrot sticks (35)

## Dinner-591 calories-chili & mixed fruit

organic black bean chili (200)

avocado (240)

watermelon (46)

## Dessert-frozen banana (105)

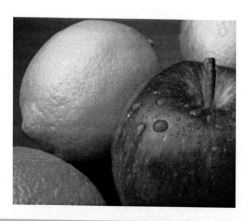

# Day 7-total 1,551 calories

Include at least 8 glasses of water = 2 with every
meal, 1 in the morning and 1 at night

## Breakfast-433 calories-egg casserole & orange juice

light multi-grain English muffin (100)

egg–1 fried (90)

slice of turkey breast (40)

garlic (15)

onions (7)

green peppers (19)

2% Swiss cheese (50)

glass of orange juice (112)

## Snack-105 calories

Banana (105)

## Lunch-413 calories-hard boiled egg, carrot sticks, smoothie

hard boiled egg (78)

carrot sticks (35)

strawberry banana smoothie (300)

## Snack #2-95 calories

apple (95)

## Dinner-511 calories-salmon, potatoes, mixed fruits & vegetables

wild caught Atlantic salmon (280)

new potatoes (60)

mixed vegetables (59)

watermelon (46)

## Reward-50 calories

dark chocolate – 1 x 9 gram piece (50)

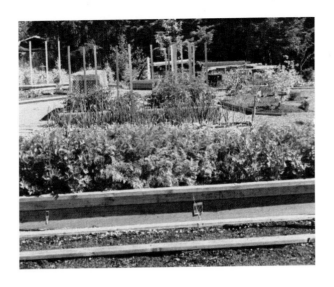

# Day 8-total 1,456 calories

Include at least 8 glasses of water = 2 with every meal, 1 in the morning and 1 at night

## Breakfast-271 calories-veggie wrap & orange juice

low carbohydrate whole wheat wrap (80)

2% low-fat Swiss cheese (50)

tomatoes (22)

onions (7)

orange juice (112)

## Lunch-494 calories-chicken salad sandwich, mixed fruits

chicken salad sandwich on whole wheat (290)

tomato slice on sandwich (5)

grapes (62)

apple (95)

raisins (42)

## Snack-105 calories

Banana (105)

## Dinner-376 calories-salmon cakes over salad, mixed fruits & vegetables

wild salmon cakes (245)

baby spinach (25)

tomatoes (22)

honeydew melon (64)

asparagus (20)

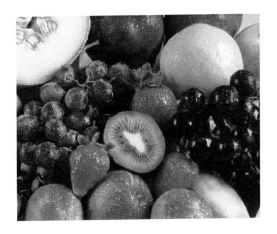

# Day 9-total 1,456 calories

Include at least 8 glasses of water = 2 with every meal, 1 in the morning and 1 at night

## Breakfast-530 calories-cereal, mixed fruits & orange juice

organic fat free milk (90)

Kashi cereal (140)

banana (105)

blueberries (83)

orange juice (112)

## Snack-140 calories

Breakfast bar (140)

## Lunch-257 calories-veggie wrap & fruit

hot veggie wrap

low carbohydrate whole wheat wrap (80)

Havarti cheese (45)

tomato (22)

onion (7)

red peppers (19)

green peppers (19)

broccoli (27)

peaches (38)

## Snack-100 calories

yogurt -low fat (100)

## Dinner-420 calories-spinach salad, wheat rolls & fruit

spinach (14)

hard boiled egg (78)

green onions (10)

tomato (22)

turkey bacon (35)

turkey breast (45)

whole wheat potato roll (80)

olive oil spread (50)

apple (95)

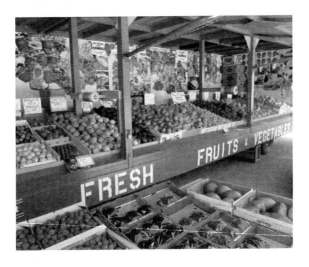

# Day 10-total 1,506 calories

Include at least 8 glasses of water = 2 with every meal, 1 in the morning and 1 at night

## Breakfast-319 calories-yogurt, mixed nuts & mixed fruits

non-fat yogurt (80)

mixed nuts (174)

blueberries (41)

strawberries (24)

## Snack-95 calories

apple (95)

## Lunch-454 calories-chicken, fruit & cottage cheese

oven roasted chicken (310)

tomato slices (5)

tangerine (37)

2% low-fat cottage cheese (102)

## Snack-105 calories

banana (105)

## Dinner-533 calories-vegetable stew, cheese toast. mixed fruits & vegetables

vegetable stew (160)

cheese toast (150) (Swiss 50 / whole grain bread 100)

strawberries (49)

grapes (62)

cantaloupe (60)

broccoli (27) w/ parmesan (25)

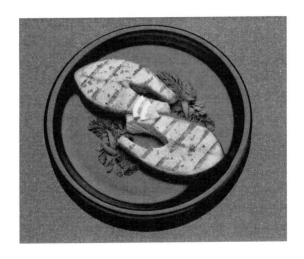

# Day 11-total 1,507 calories

Include at least 8 glasses of water = 2 with every meal, 1 in the morning and 1 at night

## Breakfast-411 calories-salmon over eggs, muffin & mixed fruits

wild salmon (280)

scrambled egg (102)

whole wheat muffin (90)

pineapple (28)

grapefruit (41)

## Snack-95 calories

apple (95)

## Lunch-430 calories-spinach & fruit salad, green beans

spinach (14)

blueberries (19)

strawberries (19)

grapes (32)

pineapple (56)

fat-free raspberry pecan dressing (50)

1 cup snap green beans (44)

## Snack-205 calories-fruit yogurt

yogurt (100)

banana (105)

## Dinner-432 calories-turkey meatloaf, fruit & vegetables

turkey meatloaf (330)

watermelon (46)

mashed cauliflower (29)

broccoli (27)

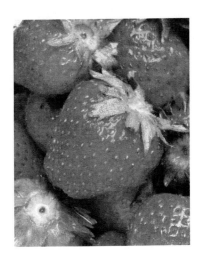

## Day 12-total 1,440 calories

Include at least 8 glasses of water = 2 with every meal, 1 in the morning and 1 at night

## Breakfast-428 calories-hard boiled egg, muffin & mixed fruits

hard boiled egg (78)

whole wheat English muffin (140)

agave nectar (60)

cinnamon (6)

grapes (32)

orange juice (112)

## Snack-105 calories

banana–1 medium (105)

## Lunch-320 calories-vegetable wrap & chips

low fat whole wheat wrap (80)

spinach (7)

radish (9)

cucumber (8)

tomato (5)

alfalfa sprouts (7)

2% low-fat cottage cheese (102)

10 pita chips (102)

## Snack-95 calories

apple–1 medium (95)

## Dinner-492 calories-spinach soufflé, fruit salad, beans, rolls

spinach soufflé (220)

fruit salad (125)

pinto beans (22)

2 whole wheat potato rolls (80)

olive oil spread (45)

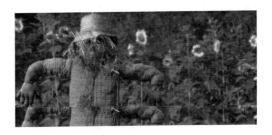

# Day 13-total 1,552 calories

Include at least 8 glasses of water = 2 with every meal, 1 in the morning and 1 at night

## Breakfast-463 calories-hard boiled egg & yogurt

hard boiled egg (78)

light fat-free yogurt (100)

1/2 cup granola on yogurt (180)

banana (105)

## Lunch-423 calories-burrito

black bean vegetable burrito (280)

salsa (36)

mango slices (107)

## Snack-95 calories

apple–1 med. (95)

## Dinner-550 calories-chicken breast, salad & mixed vegetables

roasted chicken breast (266)

fresh chopped spinach (7)

diced cucumber (8)

diced tomato (1/2 cup) (16)

diced onions (1/4 cup) (16)

mixed vegetables (237)

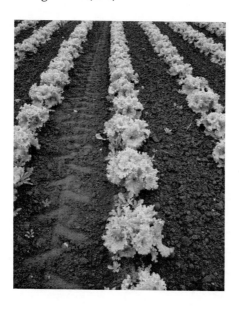

# Day 14-total 1,459 calories

Include at least 8 glasses of water = 2 with every meal, 1 in the morning and 1 at night

## Breakfast-495 calories-yogurt, mixed fruits, muffin & coffee

light fat-free yogurt (100)

grapes (32)

strawberries (27)

blueberries (41)

cantaloupe (30)

pineapple (39)

multi-grain English muffin (80)

ground cinnamon (6)

olive oil margarine–2 tablespoons (70)

10 ounce latte coffee–(70)

## Lunch-396 calories-turkey pita & apples

whole wheat pita bread (170)

light Swiss cheese (35)

alfalfa sprouts (7)

romaine lettuce (15)

tomato slices (3)

onion slices (4)

turkey breast meat (67)

apple (95)

## Snack 69 calories

10 almonds – (69)

## Dinner-449 calories-tuna, vegetables & fruit

fresh yellow fin tuna (118)

wasabi (31)

mashed cauliflower–boiled, drained w/out salt (29)

asparagus–boiled, drained w/out salt (32)

sweet potato (10)

baked apple with cinnamon (101)

## Reward-50 calories

dark chocolate – one 9 gram piece (50)

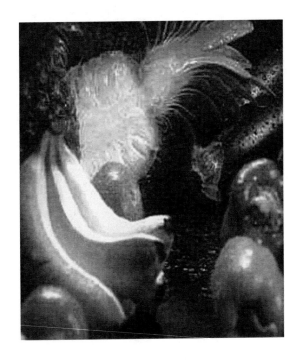

# Afterword

*O*ur prayer is that this book has been an inspiration to you and given you a few simple points that you will be able to apply to begin to live a healthier and more productive life. God has an incredible plan for every one of us. He wants us all to live a life full of abundance, but we can't sit on the couch and expect better things to fall into our lap. We need to be proactive and get up and start making changes today that will affect tomorrow. We can always come up with an excuse to slip into an old habit or not to pursue the dream or vision that God has planted in our spirit. He expects us to put forth the effort to plow the field that is required for that vision or goal that you have. Don't expect someone else to put in all of the effort for you. You have to put in the sweat equity work and then you can enjoy the harvest. In order to run and endure the race of life you need to be healthy enough to participate in the race in the first place.

It's never too late to start. You can begin with something as simple as one pound per month which if you would have started two years ago you would now be 24 pounds lighter. What about stepping up your goal to two pounds per month? That's only 1,660 calories per week or the equivalent of reducing your intake by around 240 calories each day. That's as easy as cutting out one cheeseburger, a large fry and one super-sized soda per week. If you would have started that regiment two years ago you would now be 48 pounds lighter! So where do you want to be 2 years from now? You only have yourself to blame if you don't start today. This is a brand new season for your field so start making the right decision on every seed that you sow and then watch the incredible benefits that will blossom because of your efforts. If you feel that you can't do it alone, then get a friend or relative to help you, or ask Jesus into your heart and start living every day to glorify Him. Today is the perfect day to begin to start honoring yourself. You are worthy or God wouldn't have created you in the first place. He loves you and has incredible things planned for your future.

The healthy harvest that we've talked about throughout this book isn't just for your physical health, you are constantly sowing into your own life and other's lives with almost every decision that you make. What kind of sowing are you doing while driving if you speed up and don't allow a car to get in front of you on the freeway or cut in front of someone at the grocery store to take a parking place? What kind of sowing are you doing with your language when you won't allow your children to use bad words but they hear you use them when watching a football game? You expect people at work to compliment you on a job well done, but when was the last time that you told someone how great they were and how much you appreciate them? Remember that you always reap what you sow. What kind of spouse, parent, employee, or child would you like to have? The majority of the time they are a mirror, an exact reflection of what you've sown into them. It's hard to look at a mirror sometimes because we don't always like the reflection. If other people in your life aren't reflecting what you want or had hoped for, then check your own reflection again and make sure that it resembles Jesus. If you reflect Him, then the rest doesn't matter because you are a shining light and even the darkest area can not exstinguish even the smallest light.

Start applying these sowing principles into every aspect of your life today, and one more time, read this out loud for all to hear. *I will start sowing the right seed for a healthy harvest*!

The most important decision that you can make isn't to lose weight and be healthier; it's actually to know where you will spend eternity. Has anyone ever told you that God loves you and that He has a wonderful plan for your life? We have an important question to ask you. If you were to die today, do you know for sure, beyond a shadow of a doubt, that you would go to Heaven? We'd like to share with you what the Holy Bible reads. "For all have sinned and come short of the glory of God" (Romans 3:23 KJV) and "for the wages of sin is death, but the gift of God is eternal life through Jesus Christ our Lord" (Romans 6:23 KJV). The Bible also reads, "For whosoever shall call upon the name of the Lord shall be saved" (Romans 10:13 KJV). We are all a whosoever so no one is exempt from this promise.

We're going to say a prayer for you. Lord, bless the reader of this book and their family with long and healthy lives. Jesus, make yourself real to them and do a quick work in their heart. If they have not received Jesus Christ as their Lord and Savior, we pray that they will do so now. If you would like to receive the free gift that God has for you today, say this with your heart and lips out loud. "Dear Lord Jesus, come into my heart. Forgive me of my sin. Wash me and cleanse me. Set me free. Jesus; thank you that you died for me. I believe that you are risen from the dead and that you are coming back again for me. Fill me with the Holy Spirit. Give me a passion for the lost, a hunger for the things of God and a holy boldness to preach the gospel of Jesus Christ. I'm saved; I'm born again, I'm forgiven and I'm on my way to Heaven because I have Jesus in my heart."

If you prayed that with us then we can tell you today that all of your sins are forgiven and always remember to run to God and not from God because He loves you and has a great plan for your life.[8]

Congratulations and God Bless You!

May grace and mercy follow you
all the days of your life,
Robert & Lori Evans

# Endnotes

1  UK Health Behavior Research Centre – How long does it take to form a bad habit? accessed June 6th, 2012, http://www.ucl.ac.uk/news/news-articles/0908/09080401

2  Excerpts from the FDA "Defect Levels Handbook", accessed April 27th, 2011 http://www.fda.gov/food/guidancecomplianceregulatoryinformation/guidancedocuments/sanitation/ucm056174.htm

3  Penn Metabolic & Bariatric Surgery Program– Cara Stewart, RD, LDN, accessed June 6th, 2012, http://penn-bariatric-weight-loss-surgery.blogspot.com/2011/04/eat-meals-slowly-its-worth-time.html

4  Andrade AM, Greene GW, Melanson KJ. Eating slowly led to decreases in energy intake within meals in healthy women. J Am Diet Assoc. 2008 Jul;108(7):1186-91.

5   Department of Health and Family Services State of Wisconsin, Division of Public Health, PPH 40109 (09/05)

6   Center for Disease Control,"Large Portion Sizes Have Become the New (Ab)Normal", Posted by CDC on May 21, 2012 at 9:03am http://makinghealtheasier.org/profiles/blogs/large-portion-sizes-have-become-the-new-ab-normal

7   American Heart Association, "Know Your Fats" accessed April 27th, 2011 http://www.heart.org/HEARTORG/Conditions/Cholesterol/PreventionTreatmentofHighCholesterol/Know-Your-Fats_UCM_305628_Article.jsp

8   Revival Ministries International, P.O. Box 292888 • Tampa, FL 33687, (813) 971-9999 • www.revival.com